# fat yoga

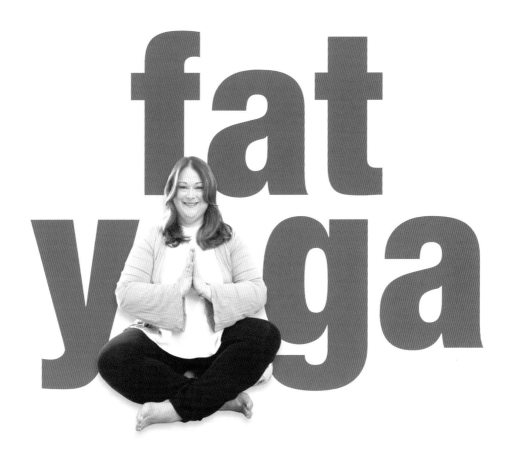

# fat yoga

## YOGA FOR ALL BODIES

SARAH HARRY

NEW
HOLLAND

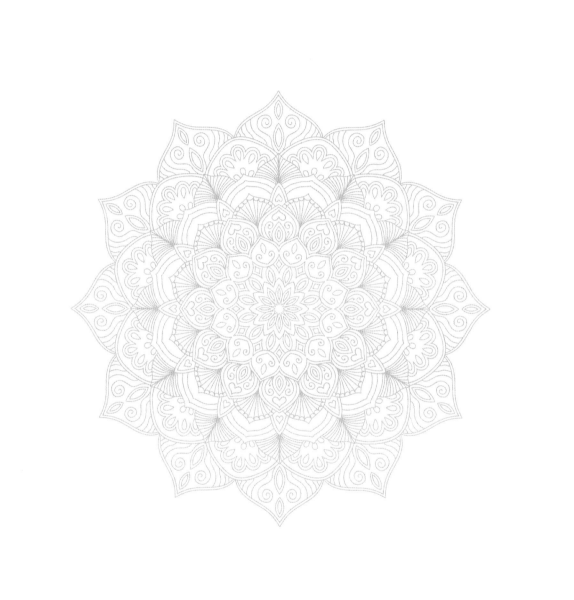

# CONTENTS

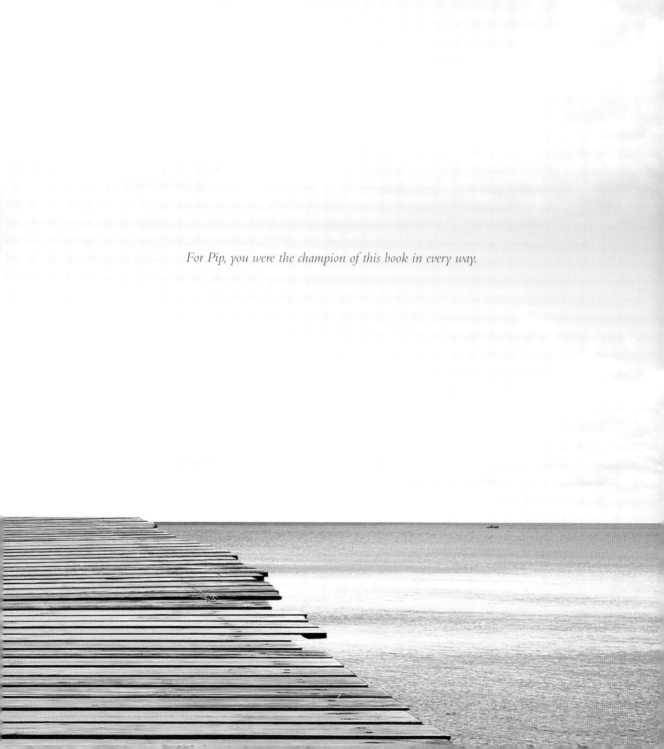

*For Pip, you were the champion of this book in every way.*

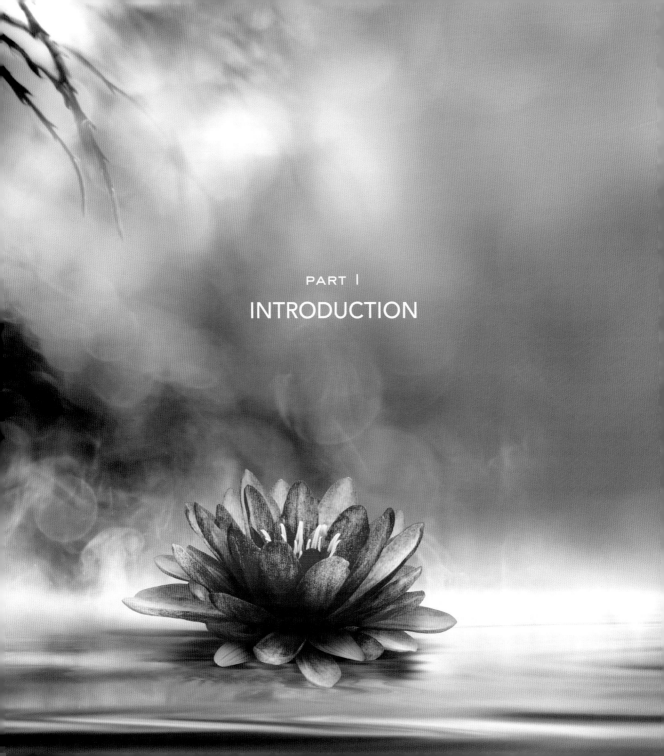

PART I

INTRODUCTION

# CHAPTER I

# WHY FAT YOGA?

*There is no wrong way to have a body.*
Glenn Marla

## WHY DID YOU CALL IT FAT YOGA?

So, once upon a time, the word 'fat' was not one I was friendly with. In fact, it was the worst and most hurtful (devastating really) word you could call me. It had greater power than any other word and I spent vast sums of money and equally silly amounts of time trying to outrun it. If it was even whispered near me my eyes would fill up and I would retreat to carrot sticks and steamed chicken, completely crushed.

My world was a complex prison of numbers for more than 20 years. I counted grams, calories, kilograms and minutes till I could eat again. I was obsessed with being lighter and the concept that it would be my golden ticket. When I took up less space I would have more: more love, more beauty, more fun, and more success.

As I found yoga I moved out of my prison of numbers to see my body for what it was. Bigger, taller and stronger than most, I wasn't going to take up less space, not ever. All that meant that somewhere along the way I had to stop running from the word 'fat' and just see it for a descriptor of my body. I had to strip it of its power over me and not allow it to hurt me. Yoga taught me to come home to my body.

Yoga is an inclusive and beautiful practice, bringing together many elements which have nothing to do with the size of your thighs or the brand of your pants. It doesn't matter if you can touch your toes or you haven't seen them for years; yoga has something to offer you.

In Fat Yoga we don't see the postures as something we need to squeeze our bodies into, in fact the postures need to fit us. In this practice we honor and respect the body, meeting it where it is. In this version of yoga size doesn't matter.

Fat Yoga completely rejects the idea that the modern 'yoga body' is the only body able to practice yoga (slender, youthful, bendy, white and able bodied) — a dangerous and unhelpful construct that adds to the pressure people currently feel to adhere to a narrow, idealized form of beauty. There is an abundance of diversity in our society, and I would like to embrace and respect those differences, not try and squeeze myself into someone else's idea of beauty.

And if you don't like my fat legs in lycra, it's very simple — just look away. I no longer care. It's my body and my business.

## WHY WE NEED FAT YOGA

Those of us in bigger bodies are often made to feel uncomfortable, visible or incompetent in traditional yoga studios and I wanted to offer a space where people could feel comfortable. It would be really great if people didn't call fat people exercising names or come up and congratulate us (both really horrible experiences), but they do.

I have been publicly humiliated, shamed, told to 'come back tomorrow when the beginners' class is on' and just not made to feel welcome in some studios. The assumptions made about me, my experience and my fitness have been breathtaking. I knew other people were struggling with this too and I wanted to bring this beautiful practice into spaces where that would never happen.

There are very few places where bigger people can exercise with ease and comfort in a class and with a teacher who understands their body and can cater to their needs, so that is why I started this movement. We need the tools to understand our bodies and how they are different but just as capable, and teachers who are welcoming and skilled to help us.

## THE GUIDING PRINCIPLES OF FAT YOGA

» All bodies can practice yoga
» All bodies deserve care
» All bodies deserve respect
» All bodies have value
» Fat Yoga will meet your body where you are physically comfortable
» Fat Yoga is a Fat Positive practice
» Fat Yoga is a body positive practice (no one body is better than another)

## AND THE REALLY IMPORTANT STUFF THAT YOU WERE TOO AFRAID TO ASK!

» You don't need to know your asana from your elbow, you can still enjoy yoga (even if you just come for the nap at the end)
» Try not to beat yourself up if your body doesn't look or move the way you want it to right now; you may surprise yourself with a regular practice
» Come with what you have. It's all you need.
» No, you're not too old. Or too inflexible!
» You don't have to be a vegan to practice yoga (I'm not! Some are!)
» Some yogis drink wine (if they want to — I do!)
» You can wear what you want and there are lots of places to buy amazing activewear for curves if you would like to (there is a list on my website)
» It's OK to cry in the lying down parts. It may not ever happen (don't panic) but sometimes when you get still and quiet, the emotions come. It's all good.
» Yoga is not a religion. Nope, no way, not at all!
» If you want it to be, it can be spiritual
» What on earth does 'namaste' mean? It's just a greeting and a farewell with your hands at your heart, but here is a lovely translation:

*Namaste*
*I honor the place in you*
*in which the entire universe resides.*
*I honor the place in you*
*which is of love, of light, of truth and of peace.*
*When you are in that place in you*
*and I am in that place in me.*
*We are one.*

## WHO IS THIS BOOK FOR?

Anyone who would like to learn or deepen their existing practice of yoga and who doesn't feel at home in a studio class or doesn't have one nearby

Anyone who would like to understand how to adapt classic postures for their body

Yoga teachers whose training didn't include teaching yoga for bigger bodies and who would like to learn how to be more inclusive in their teaching.

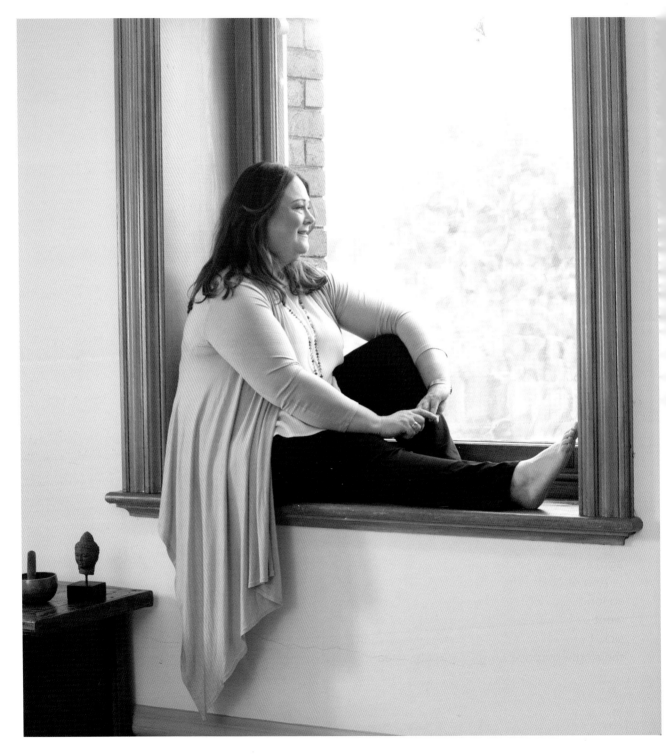

# CHAPTER 2

# MY JOURNEY

I was born in Melbourne but we traveled all over the world with my dad's work and I hopped in and out of half a dozen primary schools. Despite once pretending to be blind on the eve of one big move (ah, long story), I loved it. I felt different and special. I have always loved to travel, I was an exchange student in Virginia and a backpacker for years; from Guatemala to the outer banks of North Carolina, and I have been to some incredible places. I rode trains and planes, buses, a camel and a donkey. I have had adventures that will keep me (and my friends) entertained for years. I have always been fearless and I definitely took risks. My parents believed we could do anything we wanted and they told us that over and over. I have always had a sense of self about my work and who I am, but there was also something in the background, holding me back.

I was put on my first diet at nine and used to go to sleep wishing to wake up with thinner thighs, which would magically transform me from the girl 'who had such a pretty face' to the real deal. I was a dedicated dieter for two decades and I was at war with my body. We weren't friends. Not at all.

I never trusted my body; I didn't listen to it or its wisdom. I ignored hunger and fullness, I only moved it to burn calories and I worshiped at the altar of every single diet around. I ordered illegal diet drugs on the internet when it still made that dial-up sound, I sent away for Oprah's cookbook, I swallowed every pill, drug, potion and program I could get my hands on. I endured plastic surgery (smaller breasts) and weight loss surgery (twice, more than 15 years ago) and yet still I couldn't outrun my genes.

And of course it did work, for a while, but just like holding my breath, I could only do it for so long before I had to eat again. I thought I was weak, stupid and a failure. So the numbers went up and down, up and down. And really, although I thought I was fine, I was actually so sick. I was starving, malnourished and in chronic pain from the surgeries gone wrong. All for the single purpose of weighing less. Heartbreaking.

I struggled with an eating disorder for a decade, which I refused to speak to my parents (who took to leaving notes about it) or any professional about and I staged a fake recovery to get everyone off my back, and that worked for quite a few years. I attended an all-girls school, which was rife with a tangible fear of fat and competition, which did nothing to shift my obsession with numbers and sizes, driving me deeper into an unhappy relationship with food and eating.

I went on to university, still deeply unwell, and the culture of the residential colleges just added to my desire to be thinner and thinner. I hid my depression and eating disorder so well it just became a way of life; one person in public, another in private. At the first opportunity I packed up and moved to London.

My twenties were a blur of planes and fabric swatches as I turned a freakishly lucky encounter over gin and tonics in a genteel London suburb into a full-blown career in high fashion. There was the dinner at a royal home and the drug dealers who lived next door and the year I went to the same gym as Mick Jagger. Summers on the Italian Riviera and a brief and unsuccessful foray into plus-size modeling were all part of a time in my life where I still wasn't happy with myself, but I was happy with where I had landed. I made lifelong friends and jumped on trains with my backpack and my beaten up copy of Robert Frost's poetry for company. So many things were good.

A brief romance with an MI5 contender meant he had to list me on an official document as someone he had been out with, which led directly to me being investigated by the British immigration department. They quickly unearthed that I was not in fact working in a pub like all my friends, but was working for a fashion company which regularly took me to Milan, making it impossible for me claim I wasn't working in a 'career' job, and totally blowing the requirements of my holiday visa. They gave me three weeks to leave the country.

I had a pretty soft landing back home, securing the job in Melbourne that 'a million girls would kill for', working for Valentino. I lived on salad and ciggies and thought that $500 for a T-shirt was a bargain. A pain in the arse with a clothing allowance and a travel budget. There are some classic shots somewhere of me posing for a mag in front of my '$40,000 wardrobe' (I wish I was kidding!).

At 27 I caught sight of a photo of that nine-year-old girl and I sucked in my breath. She didn't look fat. She just looked normal. I don't know why that jarred me so much, but it completely floored me. I remember taking a day off work and evaluating my life. So shiny from the outside, such chaos when you scratched the surface.

I remember calling the telephone line of the Eating Disorders Foundation and asking them what to do. I thought they would tell me I wasn't thin enough to be worthy of treatment, but I was wrong. Slowly, alone and tentatively I started moving towards recovery, making appointments and joining a research trial. I didn't have enough money for private treatment and I didn't want to ask for help.

As I inched towards recovery I realized I couldn't work in fashion any more. The only thing I wanted to do was to resurrect my Arts degree and start again. I sold everything I owned, moved home to my parents (gah! Only to find them on the brink of a messy divorce with me squarely in the middle) and bought a dog called Chilli. I think I really wanted a baby, but a fluffy white puppy was something I could lavish with love.

I went back to university, became a psychotherapist (counselor) and I was pretty sure of my path. From the day I decided to seek help for my eating disorder I made a quiet promise to myself that I would work in the field and that helping even one person not live though what I did would be worth it. I was dogged in my vision, volunteering my time and living on a shoestring.

At the same time, I wandered totally by chance into a yoga class in a gym. It was only run every Saturday morning and, against all odds, I not only enjoyed the class, but it was taught by a genuine yogi who ignited in me a love of yoga, which was to endure. I think one of the reasons I kept coming back was I was reasonably good at it and, in her understated way, the teacher supported and encouraged my growing confidence in my body.

Yoga for me was part of coming home to my body and finally healing. I felt for the first time connected and at ease. I have now been practicing for nearly 20 years, not always continually, but through everything, there has been yoga. I have returned to the mat to get me through the hardest times and while it hasn't cured everything, it's been a place of comfort.

A chance meeting at a private eating disorders clinic I worked at for three weeks (long story!) turned out to be extremely fortunate as I met Fiona Sutherland, Australia's best dietitian (no, I am not biased), and we started Body Positive Australia over our kitchen tables. (I'd like to say it was over tea, but it was probably wine. Or gin). For the last 12 years we have worked together, building a tiny company which now offers retreats, therapy, dietetics, groups and professional development and training.

My grandmother told me when I was very young that I would never find a husband as I was too fat, and that had stayed with me, eating at my belief in myself, so I didn't really start dating till I was 30 (don't worry, I had lots of ill-advised flings!). And then I met someone.

He was so lovely and I was so happy. In reality, I was surprised. Surprised that anyone would love me and want to marry me. In the back of my head I thought the white picket fence and the two kids was not something I was worthy of. We moved in together and built a life. A good life, a life looking towards the future. Things were rosy, the wedding was beautiful, with our gorgeous 18-month-old baby in attendance, eating raisins.

What I didn't know filled an ocean.

At 2 am one night the phone call came: you don't know your husband, he's not who you think he is. Not only that but he has a pregnant girlfriend and a double life. I remember thinking that night, 'this is what it feels like to have your life crash down around your ears'. I was not the only one in shock. He fooled everyone. Everyone was reeling. Slowly and painfully all the details came to light. I felt frozen; I didn't know what to do.

You hear these stories and it seems impossible. How could I not have known? How stupid must you have to be? It's remarkable really, the level of deception that has to occur to pull off something like what he did to me. He would lovingly tell me to have a rest and he would walk our newborn to the park, I would think to myself how kind he was. Meanwhile, at the park his girlfriend would meet him for a stroll with our son.

I contacted her and she sent me every last detail down to the photographs, which was a blessing and a curse. She told me every single thing and that there were many others, not just her. It's not the sort of email you can unread. Eventually I burnt it just so when I was low I didn't pull it out and read it again, opening up the wounds.

What I later came to understand was that I was traumatized, and I had a two-year-old, so I let him come back home and I pretended it was all OK. It wasn't. We had another baby; a much loved and wanted baby who didn't sleep. And then the wheels fell off for the final time.

With no sleep, a newborn, a three-year-old and a marriage coming apart I went back to work as a counselor three weeks after my second son was born (premature, no less), trying to outrun my shambles of a life. The first time I asked for help was a request to the pediatrician to send me and my son to sleep school, which he did, reluctantly.

My husband visited me at sleep school and the nursing staff overheard him and how he spoke to and treated me and they confronted me. He was banned from the hospital, and that is what it took to realize how he treated me wasn't OK. I thought it was my fault; I was difficult and I needed to change.

At sleep school I had to face that everything was not OK and had not been for years. On some level, before then I knew it wasn't right. Over the years we were together I packed my car twice in the middle of the night and loaded my youngest child into it and drove to my mum's. She never knew; he never knew. I never went inside, I just drove home and unpacked again. I told no-one. The shame crushed me into silence.

The staff didn't want me to return home, so they held me as long as they could and they transferred me to a mother and baby unit at a private psychiatric hospital. I kept asking them what to do, but no-one would tell me; eventually I realized it was a decision nobody could make but me.

I went into a psychiatric hospital for the first time with my son with me and I thought I was going for a few days. We were there six weeks and I had three admissions in total. Without my mother, who looked after my eldest son, I wouldn't have been able to go in, and if I didn't go in I don't know if I would have survived. I am so grateful for her support, then and now.

I overdosed on a pretty lethal mix of alcohol and prescription medication on one of my visits home, after a very bad session with the relationship counselor. Back to hospital. I remember calling my family to tell them what I had done and I didn't sugar-coat any of it. I didn't want to die, but I didn't want to live either. So, that's what rock bottom looked like. Not that pretty. I feel like I can say now that I will never allow myself to go back there.

Slowly I came back to health. I returned home and, after the third and final stay in what I affectionately call the nuthouse, I made a decision. I could see that I could spend my life in and out of that very comfortable place. And with all my heart, I didn't want my children to grow up with a mother who wasn't present and was in and out of hospital.  I knew what I had to do. I took the medication, I did intensive therapy, I really learned to look after myself and I still do now. What remains is an underlying anxiety, which will never really go away, but I know how to live with. Yoga and meditation help me, but they couldn't do it all. I felt bad, as a yogi, for taking medication. During teacher training I even stopped. I think that put me back a year. So now it's all about balance!

The day after my youngest son turned one I was well enough to leave our house; the one I thought I would raise my children in, the one I loved so much. But I asked myself the question everyone does: why did I wait so long? I didn't think I could afford it and I didn't think I could cope. But I did both. The first night in my new rental property I cried a kind of messy, happy tears. I felt free and more like myself than I had in years. I remember eating toast and it tasting like the most delicious thing I had ever eaten in my now safe life, with my children sleeping nearby.

I pulled the threads of my life together and roared into my forties dating up a storm (bet you've never met an urban vampire!) and got my yoga on. In my local, suburban class I vividly remember asking my teacher, 'Sarasvati', if she thought I could be a yoga teacher? She didn't even pause, and answered, 'Yes'. At that time I didn't think it was remotely possible; there were no fat yogis in Australia and barely any overseas, nothing like the visibility and social media presence there is now.

I started looking into yoga teacher training, something I never thought I could do (surely I was much too fat) and nearly didn't follow through with it as one yoga school was horrible to me on the phone, telling me they didn't think I had what it would take. When I finally applied somewhere else I was sure they wouldn't let me in! The pure fear I felt the day I had to attend my first teacher-training intensive was enormous, I felt like someone was going to tap me on the shoulder and ask me to leave. But the opposite happened; they were lovely, inclusive and supportive. So I became a yoga teacher after a year of training. A fat one. At 40.

At first I found it really hard going creating any traction and often just one or two people showed up to classes I started in other people's studios, at awkward times of day they didn't use! But slowly a core group of yogis came and stayed (you know who you are and I love you so much!). In reality, though, it was years of hard work before anyone was interested in what I was doing. I came so close to giving up so many times!

Now my passion and privilege is about creating safe spaces for all bodies to practice and access yoga and using yoga to heal people's relationship with their body. On so many occasions I was made to feel out of place, not enough or just too fat to practice in a general studio class. This book is for anyone who feels that way to use so they can create a home practice, reconnect with their bodies and start to become more at home in their body.

After all, your body is the most incredible thing you will ever own and the most important relationship you will ever have.

# Chapter 3

# YOGA BASICS

*Yogas citta vrtti nirodhah.*
*Yoga is the stilling of the movement in the mind.*
Patanjali, Sutra 1:2

## WHAT IS YOGA?

For the first 15 years of my yoga practice I literally had no idea of the history of yoga! I just showed up to class and smiled and nodded when the teacher used Sanskrit (what the hell was that?) and talked vaguely about yogic concepts. It's actually amazing I practiced for so long, absorbing so little (this was a real drawback at yoga teacher training) so here is a little bit of yoga history for you so you can hold your own at dinner parties!

I really did think it was about how good I was at touching my toes (pretty good it turned out; a completely irrelevant detail) but it is so much more. Yoga is an ancient practice, about 4000 years old and first passed from teacher to student in an oral tradition. About 2000 years ago the Indian sage Patanjali committed 196 'sutras' to parchment, outlining the 8 limbs or parts of yoga and the basis of all the yoga we know and practice today. Of these 196 sutras or seeds of wisdom, only a couple refer to the 'asanas' or movements in yoga and the rest delve deeply into the other 7 limbs. Traditionally, the physical yoga we are so familiar with in modern yoga was just a vehicle to prepare the body to sit for meditation.

I was trained in hatha yoga (classical yoga), a tradition that comes directly from the wisdom of Patanjali and all the ancient sages. In my teaching we follow no specific lineage or guru, instead seeking to learn from all the great teachers, ancient and modern.

## THE EIGHT LIMBS OF YOGA AS OUTLINED BY PATANJALI (200 AD)

1. Yamas (ethical considerations, how we conduct ourselves in life)
2. Niyamas (self-observation and discipline)

3. Asana (the physical movements of yoga, what most of modern studio yoga resembles!)
4. Pranayama (the breath)
5. Pratyahara (the withdrawal of your senses)
6. Dharana (concentration)
7. Dhyana (meditation)
8. Samadhi (the attainment of bliss or peace)

Everyone's journey is different in yoga. Many are attracted to the physical benefits and aren't drawn to the spiritual side of the practice. I invite people to learn at their own pace and if the spiritual (and, importantly, secular) ignites some curiosity in you, then I encourage you to seek more knowledge. It's up to you to construct your own practice with the parts that feel relevant to you. Even if you just like the stretching and the napping. That's fine too!

## EMBODIMENT AND JOYFUL MOVEMENT

It took me years to move towards either of these concepts! My experience is that not everyone likes to move or exercise. I was that girl who would cry the night before school running carnivals. You know the one, the largest, slowest and all round physically hopeless one. So I was either being coerced into 5 am rowing training (I was abysmal) or I was huddled in a corner of the gym trying to make my fat 'cry', or some such concept sold to me by whatever diet I was giving my money to that month. I still don't see myself as a 'natural' and some days (weeks?), let's face it, it's an effort to roll out my mat, but over time I have realized that there is a joyful opportunity to move for everyone.

So many of us live our lives with a strong inner critic, operating almost exclusively in our heads and it's so, so easy to listen to the voice that we aren't good enough or someone else is better. The reason most people don't go to yoga? Mostly people tell me it's fear. Fear of being the oldest, least flexible or biggest. So for some of us we need to push back decades of conditioning to even show up on our mat. Yay! Good job!

Yoga helps move our attention and our experience of living into the body. Embodiment is connecting with a sense of ease in our bodies. Experiencing all our sensations, without judgment (where we can). It is valuing and being comfortable in our skins. If I had to nominate the thing which most of my clients with body image issues would like, it is 'to be comfortable', and I believe yoga helps us achieve that.

Joyful movement is a wonderful part of life. The beauty of the yoga practice is that it can be tailored to you. And remember, yoga is not just movement; you are still practicing when you are meditating or practicing pranayama (breathing exercises).

## WHAT ARE THE BENEFITS OF A YOGA PRACTICE?

*Yoga is like music: the rhythm of the body, the melody of the mind, and the harmony of the soul create the symphony of life.* BKS Iyengar

I have seen a lot of these lists! They often have very magical and physiologically impossible things on them! I am sorry, but you can't detox via the yoga twists. We have kidneys and a liver for that. But it's worth knowing that there are many, varied benefits to a yoga practice.

**Physical benefits**
» Increased flexibility
» Increased mobility
» Greater muscle strength
» Better at sex (HA! Just to see if you are paying attention!)
» Reduced stress hormones
» Improved balance
» Stronger bones
» Improved cardiovascular health
» Improved posture
» Greater respiratory function
» Improved back pain
» Reduced tension in the muscles
» May improve sleep
» Some postures reduce heart rate and blood pressure

**Psychological benefits**
» May assist with anxiety
» May assist with depression
» Lowers stress levels
» Helpful in improving body image
» Increases concentration
» May assist with eating disorder recovery
» May assist with brain function
» Helps in regulating your adrenal function (reducing cortisol)

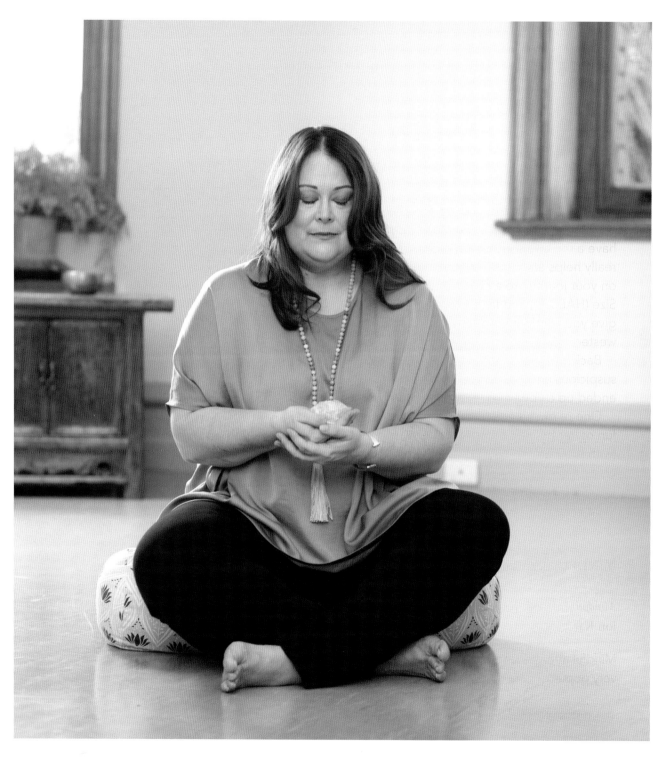

# CHAPTER 4

# FINDING BODY PEACE

Over the years I have noticed the effect yoga has on body image and after years of treating people I now use the words 'body peace' to describe what people really seek. They want to have a more relaxed and peaceful relationship with their body. Yoga and joyful movement really helps and I have identified a few modern and ancient ideas which I think will help you on your journey to a peaceful body image. Mindfulness, self-compassion, Health At Every Size (HAES ™) and fat activism are all pieces of the puzzle, to enrich your practice and maybe give you a little bit more to think about off the mat. These themes are from yogic wisdom and western science, two things I love to blend together!

Back in the distant past I used to believe the yogic wisdom was a little bit hippie and suspicious and not for me. There is a bit (a lot?) of faint amusement from my friends that I ended up a yoga teacher and, let's face it, a believer in chakras.

One of my friends is a Reiki master and had to suffer many years of me mercilessly making fun of her beliefs, mostly because I was a bona fide unbeliever in anything I couldn't see (with the exception of weight loss miracles!) for most of my twenties. I am not sure when that changed, but I know yoga played a part. It made sense to me to start to believe in subtle layers of experience which couldn't be seen or quantified, only felt. What a hippie I am now! I even wear mala beads and chant (making me ultra-spiritual, of course!).

## MINDFULNESS

*Mindfulness means paying attention in a particular way; on purpose, in the present moment and non-judgmentally.*
Jon Kabatt-Zin

Mindful attention is a key part of the yoga practice. While the practice of mindfulness is currently very popular in the West, it is an ancient part of the wisdom traditions like yoga and Buddhism.

You will often hear me say in the beginning of a class, 'just allow yourself to settle here on your mat in this present moment'. I like to encourage mindful pauses in classes where you let the effects of the practice settle over you. I find in many faster classes there is a tendency to rush from one posture to the next without actually feeling how the previous one made your body feel. I encourage people to slow and stop and feel into the yoga rather than mindlessly following my instructions.

We are only just beginning to understand the ways in which mindfulness enriches our experience of the world and can change our brain for the better! It has completely changed my experiences of living. I used to move so fast I missed almost all the detail of life. Now I practice mindfully both formally and informally; I slow, I breathe and I am present for my life.

There is a modern tendency to simplify mindfulness to just 'be in the moment' but it is much more than that.

**Mindfulness is:**
» Observing what is happening in our bodies and minds from moment to moment
» Not being judgmental or critical about our experiences
» Being curious about our experiences
» Accepting what is happening now

**Mindfulness helps us with:**
» Embodiment (moving away from just a 'shoulders up' experience of life)
» Increasing our levels of body trust
» Improving our relationship to our body
» Learning complexities of appetite
» Dealing with difficult thoughts
» Dealing with difficult feelings
» Slowing the overactive mind
» Decreasing anxiety
» Increasing the time between thought and action
» Changing the brain and rewiring neural pathways
» Living a richer more meaningful life

## AHIMSA AND SELF-COMPASSION

*If your compassion does not include yourself, it is incomplete.* Jack Kornfield

A key part of yoga philosophy is the concept of ahimsa, which is a Sanskrit word which means non-violence or non-harming. Importantly, this means not harming others, but also being kind and compassionate towards ourselves.

I feel like I am skilled at this now, but it's been like developing strength in a muscle, I have just used repetition to make it so! My inner critic used to be merciless. I tore myself down at every opportunity. It prevented me from doing so many things: 'you are too fat to wear that, go there, talk to that person'. I listened so closely to all the horrible things my mind said. Now I just see those thoughts and let them pass on by. I have things to do and life to live!

Developing ahimsa is a key part of self-compassion, which has been recently adapted and researched extensively in the West.

A yoga practice encourages you to hear the critical voice when it emerges and to be compassionate. We often find it easy to be kind to our friends and family but speak to ourselves so critically. Yoga asks that you lean a little closer to being kinder to yourself, understanding you aren't perfect and accepting where you are in the present moment. Even just in that breath, just for a moment.

The practice of self-compassion has become so important to my teaching of yoga; I try and weave it into each and every class so people get used to the idea of 'kindfulness' and can begin to imagine being compassionate to themselves when previously they had only ever been critical.

For some people this can be a radical shift, so take your time and start slow. In a moment of difficulty or struggle (on or off the mat) take your hand and place it on your heart and remind yourself 'things are tough right now, and I am doing what I can'.

Kristen Neff, a self-compassion researcher and writer divides self-compassion into a very simple model.

**Self-compassion comprises three separate but interconnected ideas:**
» Mindfulness (being aware in the present moment of when we are having a hard time without being judgmental or harsh towards ourselves)
» Common humanity (you are not alone in your experiences, everyone has tough times and

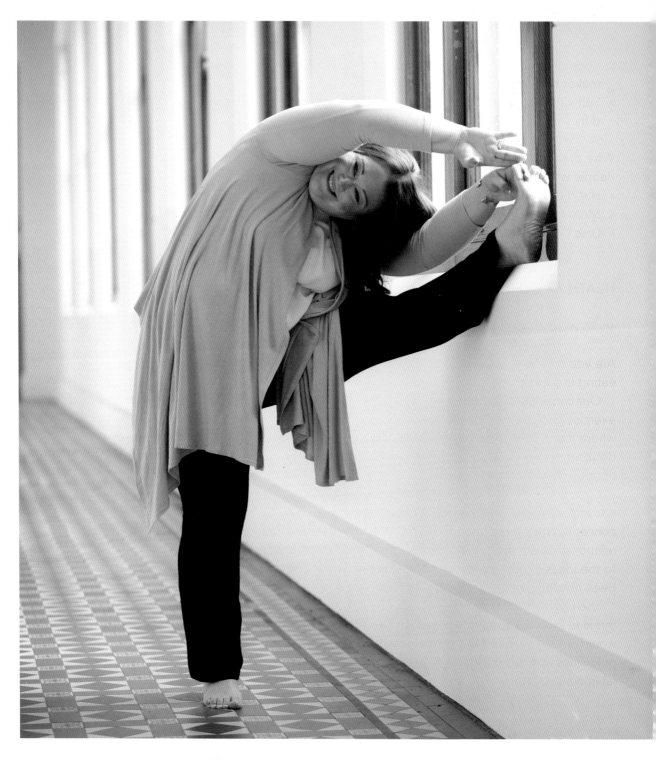

makes mistakes, no-one is perfect)
» Self-kindness (speaking and acting with kindness towards ourselves when things are difficult, much as you would a friend)

**Why practice self-compassion?**
People who practice self-compassion have been shown to be:
» Happier
» More optimistic
» Less likely to experience anxiety and depression

## HEATH AT EVERY SIZE (HAES)™ AND NON-DIET APPROACHES

*You can't tell how healthy someone is just by looking at them.* Sarah Harry

Are you constantly thinking about the next diet (Monday of course!) or restricting your food or eating in some punitive way? Then the HAES movement is for you!

Our current society is obsessed with weight and making your weight and food and exercise choices moral reflections of who you are as a person. We are now in a crazy time where if you drink a green smoothie you are a better person than the person next to you drinking the chocolate one! I call this 'buying a health halo' and it's a really unhelpful view of nourishment.

I first came across the 'non-diet' approach through meeting the pioneering Dr Rick Kausman and reading his book *If not dieting, then what?* and it was like a revolutionary concept (highly recommended!). You don't have to diet. You can have a respectful relationship with food, eating, movement and your body. I was stunned. Had I been exposed to the ideas of how futile weight-loss dieting was (with a failure rate of 95–98 %) it would have been revolutionary to me and, I think, prevented many years of pain.

There is literally no other medical advice given so frequently in our health system today with this kind of low success rate (less than 5% of people permanently lose weight via dieting). It would not be tolerated in any other treatment plan, so it just amazes me that so many of our guidelines and recommendations still push for weight-loss dieting. I think the entrenched fear of fat in our society has a lot to do with this, something I would dearly love to see shift.

All my classes are body-positive zones, with no number or diet talk to support this approach, and it's a core part of my clinical work helping people heal their relationship with food, eating and body image.

HAES principles advocate that a focus on healthy behaviors, rather than a focus on reducing body size, is the most useful way to support people of all sizes to take care of their health. I believe health is multifaceted and also includes things like mental health, social connection and happiness! Making it all about a number is a very narrow, unhelpful and limiting view. I also believe that you don't owe anyone health and no-one has any obligation to embrace any health behavior. Your body and your health are your business.

## FAT ACTIVISM AND POSITIVITY

*#LoseHateNotWeight.* Virgie Tovar

I don't know if I would have had the courage to embrace the word 'fat' and put myself and my body 'out there' so to speak if not for the fat activist movement and the attention the men and women of this movement have brought to the fact that fat people are regularly stigmatized and discriminated against. Their voices, social media presence, articles, books and even TED talks have empowered me to be able to own and embrace my fat body even more.

Many fat people in my classes have been the victims of nasty bullying, trolling and discrimination. This has a significant toll on people, another reason I feel that safe spaces to be with other fat people, free from discrimination, are important.

I listened quietly in the background in the early years, reluctant to really embrace the word or the movement. In some ways I wish I had found it sooner, but I wasn't ready. The shame held me back and now the shame is gone.

The fat activist movement is a social and political movement which seeks to change and challenge the stigma and discrimination that people living in larger bodies regularly receive. There is now significant evidence in the research that larger people are regularly discriminated against in areas such as the workplace and in healthcare (just two examples of many). The fat acceptance movement believes that all bodies have equal value and that there is a need to advocate for the rights of people of size.

While we struggle with many areas of bias and discrimination in our society, I believe that it is critical not to make judgments about people based on size or weight. Stigmatizing one type of body as 'bad' or less healthy is a very narrow view of health, serves no-one and harms a lot of people. The fat activist movement believes that fat is not a slur, simply a descriptor and seeks to reclaim the word fat as an empowering change in semantics. I certainly was not the first to use the word 'fat' in a positive way; that shift comes directly from the fat activist movment.

Some people have been uncomfortable with the name 'Fat Yoga' and this has not been body-size dependent, as some of my students tell me they are still not comfortable with it and they don't use it themselves. I can see why, as the word has so often been used as a slur, but for me we are reclaiming the word and stripping it of its negative history.

An empowering and feminist stance against the stigma and shame that bigger bodies have to endure in our culture!

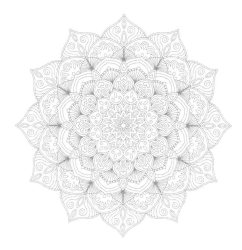

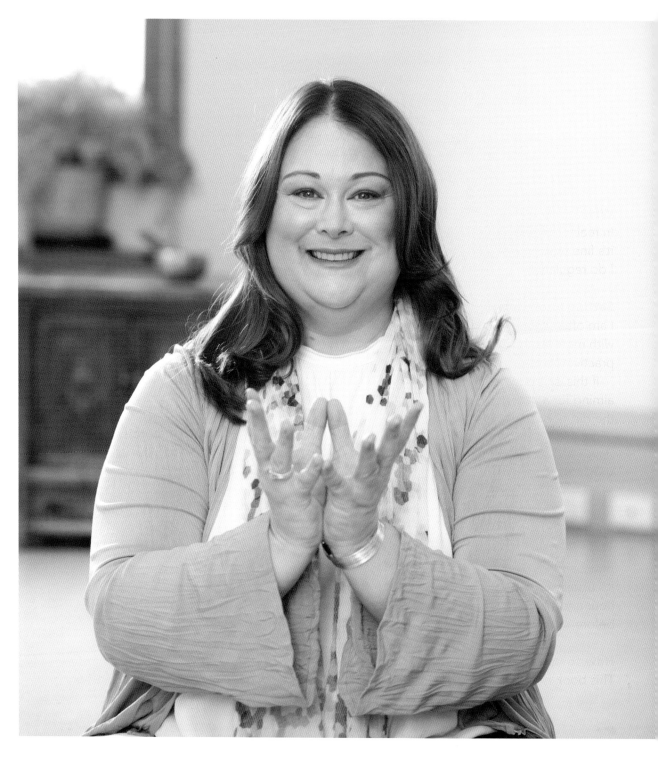

# Chapter 5

# GETTING STARTED

## WHAT DO I NEED TO GET STARTED?

In reality, not much! People often believe that they require fancy mats or expensive pants, but it's fine to just show up on a little piece of carpet in your home wearing your PJs — something I do regularly!

### Setting aside time

I am often besieged by small bodies or furry pets who enthusiastically want to practice yoga with me when I roll out my mat at home. This is fun and I love to teach them, but I prefer to practice without distractions, so I try to choose a time when I might be able to practice alone!

If this isn't possible for you (or your furry family interrupts), then that is fine too. We are aiming for a flexible and sustainable practice. The ancient yogis talked about just sweeping the dirt floor to make the practice space clean, with fresh air!

It can be difficult to have the discipline for a home practice, so I use my self-compassion skills to be flexible and understanding of myself, and my available time and energy. Some days I don't practice at all, and that is fine. If we begin our yoga journey with an expectation that we will be perfect at finding large chunks of time each day, then we may not start at all! A few minutes of mindful breathing is still yoga to me. Start small and build up your practice time!

### Food and drink

It's usually wise not to practice yoga on a full stomach. I would suggest waiting at least an hour after your last meal to make it more comfortable. I don't recommend drinking alcohol before your practice (hmm, just trust me on this one!).

### How to use this book

This book is a guide and you are welcome to dip in and out of it for what you may need on any given day. You can do the practices in the way I have outlined them or you can create your own sequences (being mindful to place stronger postures later in your practice). There is a list at the end of Part 3.

**A balanced Fat Yoga practice**
In Fat Yoga we sequence the postures in an 'arc' to support your body, so you are flowing through the practice with ease. What that means is that we start on the floor, come to knees and then standing before coming back to the floor. Most often my classes are not about jumping up and down, which many of my students find uncomfortable.

» Beginning on your back (supine)
» Seated postures
» Kneeling postures
» Standing postures
» Prone postures (on your front)
» Supine postures (on your back)
» Inverted postures (your head is lower than your heart)
» Ending with Savasana (on your back)

A classic class includes:
» Centering
» Warming up
» Pranayama (breath work)
» Back bends
» Forward bends
» Balances
» Lateral stretches
» Twists
» Inversions
» Savasana or meditation

> **A NOTE ABOUT SALUTES TO THE SUN - SURYA NAMASKAR**
>
> Salutes are often a key practice in traditional hatha yoga practices, however I don't always teach them, as my students sometimes find that going quickly from lying to standing is not as enjoyable as the 'arc' practice. I do regularly offer a 'seated salute', which eliminates that issue by staying on the floor (page 44).

## The breath/pranayama

*Breath is the bridge which connects life to consciousness, which unites your body to your thoughts.*
Thich Nhat Hanh

For a while I didn't really get the breathing thing in yoga. I think I just didn't truly understand how to do it! A teacher would explain and I wouldn't be able to connect with it. But, over the last ten years, as I struggled with a more anxious mind, I really started to understand its healing qualities. I now practice it every day (very informally), sometimes just in the car! The breath practices are in Part 3.

I struggle with a long-term anxiety disorder and I use pranayama as one of my tools to manage it, alongside yoga, medication and making sure I can get a lot of rest and good nourishment.

The study of the breath, or the breath practices, are called pranayama and, as one of the eight limbs of yoga, it is a vital part of our practice. The word itself can be divided up into two parts 'Prana', which is translated as 'life force' and 'Ayama' described as 'control', so the two together describe the art of controlling the breath.

A very simple way to honor the breath in our practice is to mindfully connect with it. I sometimes let my attention rest on my breath by repeating internally 'I am breathing in/I am breathing out', particularly when I am in the slower and more restorative postures, which helps my mind not to wander (which is what minds are designed to do!).

In yoga we traditionally breathe in and out through the nose. This tells the brain it's time to move into a more relaxed state. If this type of breathing is not possible for you for any reason, just breathe comfortably how you prefer.

Another useful tip when you are practicing alone is to note that generally we inhale as the limbs move away from the body and exhale as they draw back in.

## Setting intentions – sankalpa

*The quieter you become, the more you can hear.* Ram Dass

The Sanskrit word 'sankalpa' means to set an intention, vow or desire and in yoga we often use this at the beginning of our practice. You may bring to mind literally anything which has meaning for you so sometimes for me it will be very simple: 'I am breathing deeply' (we use the present tense when we set the sankalpa), which used to sound funny to me, but I got used to it and I think it helps!

Traditionally this is deeper than a simple target or goal, but goes to the heart of who you are and assumes that what you want or need already resides inside you. It therefore becomes important to repeat it internally to yourself in the present tense, for example 'I am kind and loving to my body' or 'I am love itself'.

Another key part is remembering or bringing to mind your sankalpa a couple of times during the class, so it stays at the forefront of your mind.

### How to discover your sankalpa
The Vedanta tradition outlines three stages:
1. Sravana, a willingness to be able to hear the message (what is your most heartfelt desire?)
2. Manana, attuning to the message and welcoming it (without judgment)
3. Nididhyasana, to do what the message requires (how do I move into helping my heartfelt desire come true?)

### Setting up the practice space
Ideally there is a small corner in your room or home where you can practice yoga. My dream house will have a little home studio for sure, but right now, with limited space, I just roll out my mat in the living room, kicking aside Lego and Shopkins as I go!

The ideal place is one in which you feel comfortable, physically and mentally, and you have the space to move around. One suggestion is to turn off devices so your full attention is on the time you have to practice.

**Optional extras!**

Music: some people like to practice to music (you can find me and my 'Restore' playlists on Spotify for some inspiration) and others prefer silence. It's completely up to you.

Aromatherapy: if you respond to particular scents you may like to burn some oil or a candle. I love both these practices, but they are not essential.

Props: I love props (the props in this book are from Stretch Now) and I feel they really help bigger bodies find ease in some postures, but you can make your own at home.

**Props**

| Prop used | Home alternative |
|-----------|------------------|
| Mat | Carpet |
| Bolster | Couch cushions |
| Block | Large books |
| Strap | Belt or scarf |
| Eye bag | Scarf |
| Chair | Chair |
| Blanket | Blanket |

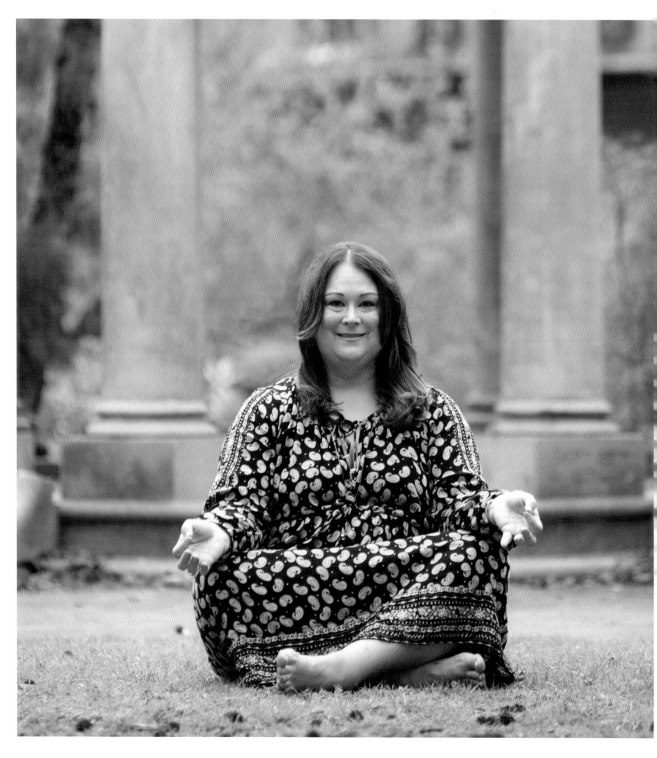

# Chapter 6

# SAFETY AND PRECAUTIONS BEFORE YOU PRACTICE

*Do not kill the instinct of the body for the glory of the pose.*
Vanda Scaravelli

## YOUR BODY, YOUR RANGE OF MOVEMENT

Everyone has an individual body with a different range of movement in each of its muscles and joints. It is very important to honor not only your body, but also its individual range. For example, you may have longer or shorter arms than the person next to you or they may have hypermobile joints or be restricted in some areas. I sometimes say in class that it's a great idea to 'keep your eyes on your own mat'!

What I first was praised for, and one of the reasons why I thought I was 'good' at yoga, is that I have a hypermobile spine. So without any trouble at all I can pop my hands flat on the ground. I used to do this often, thinking I was awesome and very yogic! But now I recognize that that isn't practice or skill, it's just an unhelpfully large range of movement, which I need to take care I don't overextend.

In studio classes, it's wise never to compare your body to anyone else's. In home practice, be mindful to use the pictures as a guide and to see which version of the posture is right for you. There is no right or wrong and for most postures there are several different ways to be comfortable. Listening carefully to where your body wants to stop and then stopping is a skill (the ego affects the best of us!).

Never push past the range that is comfortable for you. **There is no good pain in yoga.** Pain is the body's way of telling us to stop and go back to a more appropriate point. It's important to listen to it to avoid injury.

*Sometimes your wisest course is to leave out that posture (really, it's better to skip something than hurt yourself!).*

The following are some common areas of discomfort (this is a very basic list, if you have specific injuries please see your healthcare provider to make sure a yoga practice is safe for you):

**Knees**
Many people have issues with their knees and this can be worked around. Wherever there is a posture on the knees and you have an injury or tenderness in your knees you can:
1. Try padding your knees with a blanket or soft block.
2. Modify to the seated version for example Cat/Cow on pages 67–68.

**Shoulders**
In many yoga practices there is a cue to have your arms above your head. This may not suit your shoulders or may aggravate them. In place of that try:
1. Bring your arms down by your side in the standing postures.
2. Bring your hands into prayer position.

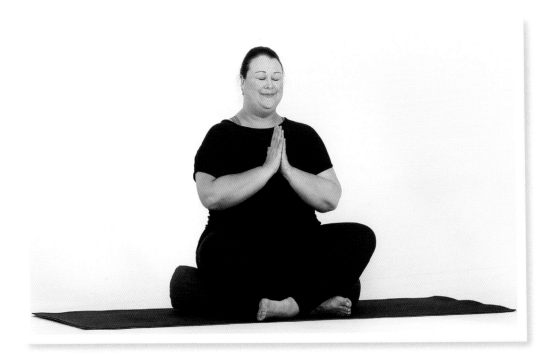

3. Where there is a cue to take your arm up toward the ceiling, like in Triangle position, just fold your arm into the small of your back, palm facing out.

## Necks
If you have a tender neck it can be good to note the following points:
1. Wherever there is a posture that asks you to 'look up' then consider just leaving that part out and keeping your gaze steady in front of you.
2. When lying on your back remember to place a folded blanket under your neck for support.

## Wrists
There are a few postures, like Downward Facing Dog, which put a lot of pressure on the wrists and shoulders and if you feel any pain:
1. The best and safest alternative is Wall Dog.

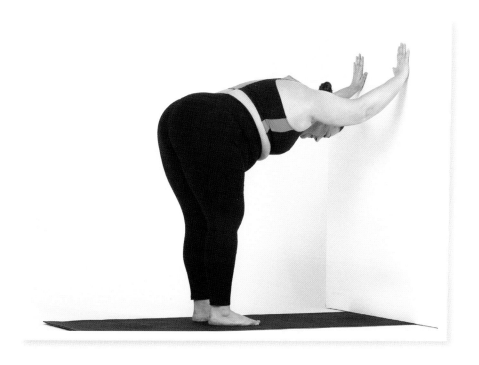

2. Sometimes with wrist issues you can try dropping down onto your forearms, if that is comfortable, to take the weight off the wrists.

3. Sometimes it helps to roll up the front of your mat an inch or two to make a little wedge to provide more support for your wrists.

**Feeling dizzy**

When we take our head down below our heart, for example in forward bends, it may make us feel dizzy if our blood pressure is higher than average. Or you may just not feel comfortable with your head down. Some alternatives are:

1. Lifting your head up in the posture may ease the issue.

2. Try using a chair or bolster, such as in the Wide Leg Forward Bend on pages 63–64.

3. Taking out any forward bends or inversions from your practice may be appropriate.

**Boobs!**

Not everyone has them and they don't bother everyone, but for some people larger breasts can get in the way of a comfortable practice or even breath, and it's never a good look to pass out during a yoga practice!

1. One option is to double up on your bras and wear two sports bras to really keep your breasts in place.

2. A second option (not for the faint hearted) is to use a scarf or yoga strap to 'bind' them down. I find the strap pretty good for this.

3. Don't practice the postures that don't allow an easy flow of breath. They aren't right for you. It's all good!

**Bellies**

Lots of people don't feel comfy about their stomachs, but whenever I feel frustrated about mine getting in the way a little (it happens) I remember what I told my son when he was little and he asked me about my tummy, 'Why is it so fat mummy?' and I just said to him, 'It's beautiful, isn't it?! And you used to live there!'

Some people find the midsection more of a hindrance than others (not always size dependent). One yoga teacher I had once said to me 'you need to make room for your abundance my dear.' (True, but not necessarily needing to be broadcast to the room!)

1. Just move to make room, so make space by widening your stance or moving your legs

further apart so that when you fold forward you have a sense of spaciousness, not cramped discomfort.

2. Move the belly. This is recommended by many fat yoga teachers, but I have had a mixed response to it personally and in classes. So experiment and see how it feels to you. Very gently and with love and respect fold your belly in towards your spine to create some more space to move. Moving or folding my belly seems to limit my breath, but everyone experiences it differently.

**Time spent in each posture**
This is a personal choice based on the time you have to practice and your energy levels or needs on the day. Generally I suggest 3–10 breaths, but feel free to adjust for your needs. Many of these postures can be made restorative in nature by holding them for longer periods. The positions that are suitable to remain in for 3–10 minutes each are *marked with a colored square.*

**Eyes open or closed?**
I know it sounds a bit crazy, but I always practice with my eyes closed when I am at home. Sometimes when I am teaching I forget where I am and close my eyes as I am so used to it! I recommend that once you get the hang of the postures and which hand goes where, close your eyes every now and then. It really helps to feel more into the body and deepen the experience.

If you don't like to close your eyes (some people don't, and that's OK) then just practice how you feel safe and comfortable!

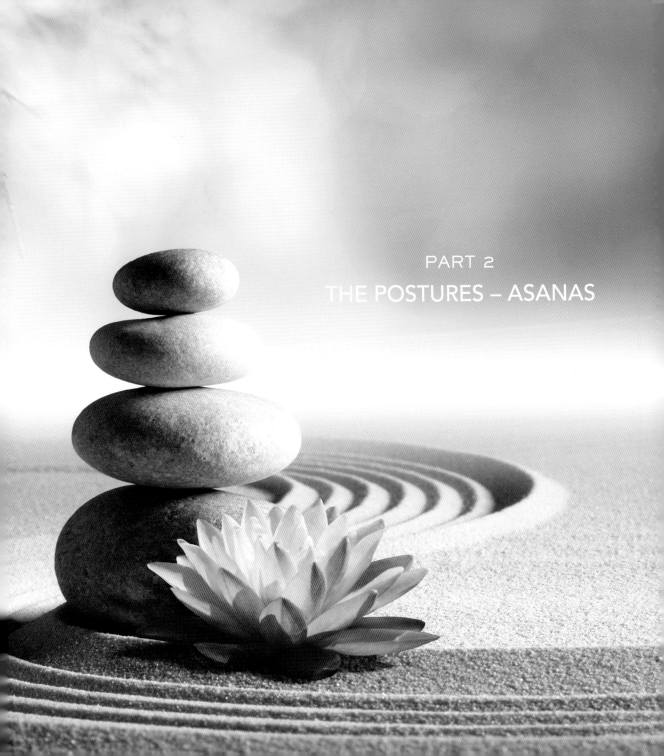

PART 2
THE POSTURES – ASANAS

## SALUTE TO THE SUN – SURYA NAMASKAR

The seated salute is a lovely warm-up, which I regularly use. If you are using it as part of your warm-up then I suggest you move slowly and be mindful of not overstretching in any of the positions, as our joints and muscles are not warm yet.

I will often practice this in the cross-legged position (and make sure I cross my legs in the opposite direction after each salute to make sure my body is evenly stretched) with a folded blanket under my hips to elevate them and keep my lower back and hips protected.

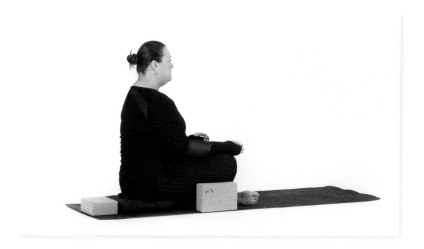

### Hints and Tips
Some of my students don't feel comfortable at all with crossed legs (I always find it funny that it's called the 'Easy Pose' when so many don't find it easy at all!). If you prefer, a very simple modification is to sit in Staff Posture (page 57) instead. Any time in yoga that you are seated on the floor, feel free to substitute your own most comfortable seated position or sit on a chair.

## Seated Salute

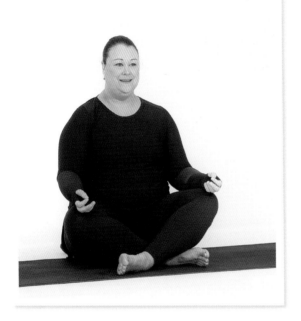

1. Sit in your most comfortable seated position and take a couple of mindful 'sigh' breaths — take a deep breath in through the nose and 'sigh' out the tension through the mouth (make as much noise as you like!).

2. Float your arms to shoulder height, imagine you are hugging the arm bones into your shoulder socket and rotate your palms to face up towards the ceiling.

3. Slowly take your arms all the way over your head, making sure your shoulders relax down away from your ears, and take a breath or two.

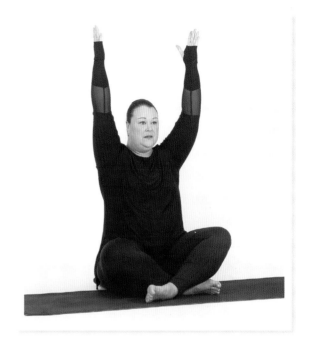

4. On the exhale, fold carefully forward, hinging from your hips, so your arms are resting on your body or on the floor in front of you and take a breath or two.

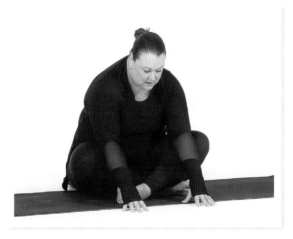

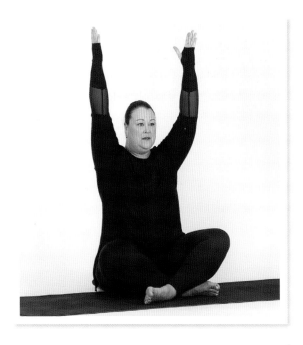

5. On the inhale, using your stomach muscles, come back up, bringing your arms up over your head.

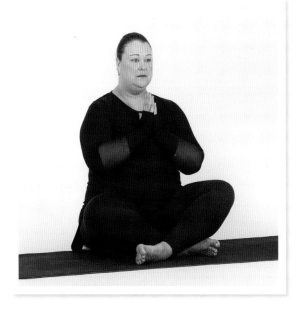

6. Exhale and bring your palms together and down through the midline of your body to Prayer position.

7. From here, take your left hand across your body to your right knee and your right hand behind you in a gentle twist, fingers resting on the floor or block, keeping your chin parallel to the floor and lifting through your chest, looking gently over your shoulder if it suits your neck. Take a few breaths here before twisting to the left side.

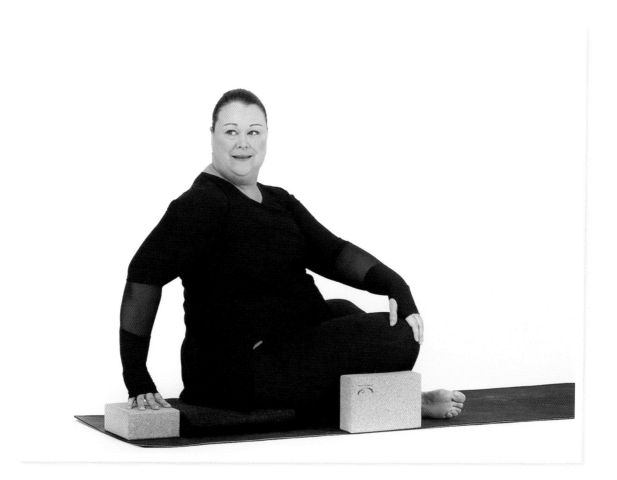

8. Return to center and take your right hand and place it on the floor next to you (in line with your hip) and then float the left hand up and over your head towards the right, palm facing down, stretching through the side body. Take a few breaths here before coming up to center and placing your left hand down to complete the stretch on the left side.

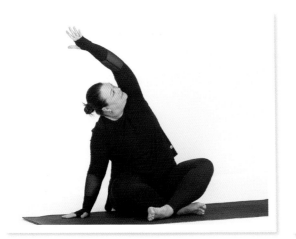 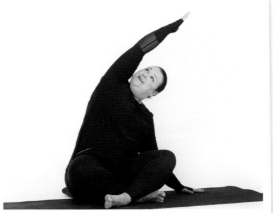

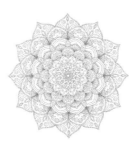

9. After a couple of rounds of this lateral stretch bring your arms back to center rotate your palms towards the ceiling and on the inhale take your arms overhead, palms facing each other.

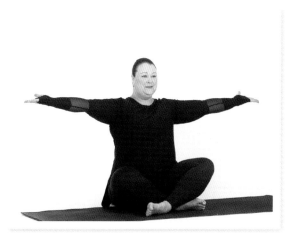 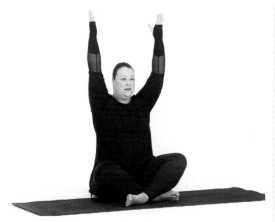

10. On the exhale breathe your hands back down the center line of the body to Prayer position.

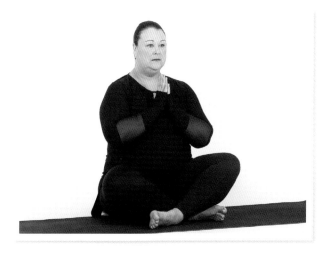

**Modified Salute**

I have modified this salute to allow for the difficulty some people find in a traditional salute (tummies and boobs can get in the way!). There is no downward facing dog, however, if you enjoy it feel free to add it in.

Sun Salutes can be a great way to add some movement to your practice as they incorporate many elements of a yoga practice into a simple vinyasa (flowing set of movements), however they don't suit everyone.

Sometimes if I am low on energy I will choose the salute, but do it really slowly and stay in each posture for a luxurious amount of time, with my attention on my breath.

The important thing to remember is that it's your practice; you decide what you need on any given day!

**Hints and Tips**

There is always the option to widen your legs more than hip width apart when practicing the forward bends to make room for your body.

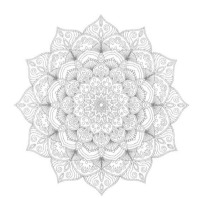

1.  Begin in Mountain Posture with your hands in Anjali Mudra (Prayer Position) and take a few full breaths.

2.  Slowly take your arms up over your head on the inhale and bring the palms together.

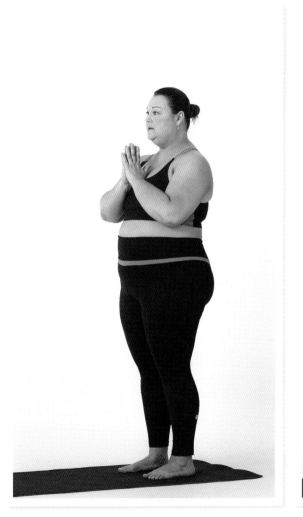

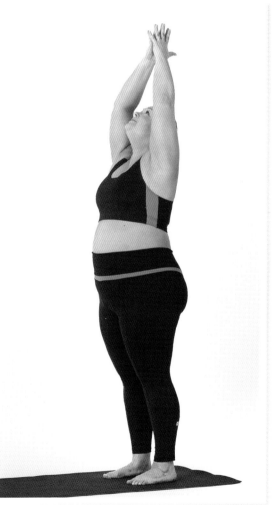

3. On the exhale take the arms out to the side as you fold forward from your hips into a forward bend (a soft bend in the knees can feel great here).

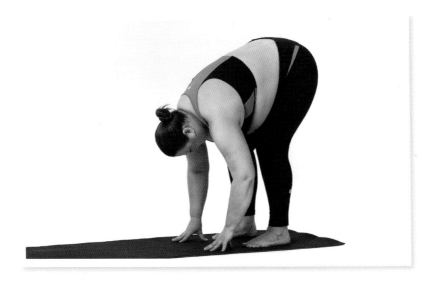

4. Bend your knees deeply and drop your hands and then knees gently to the floor into Tabletop Position.

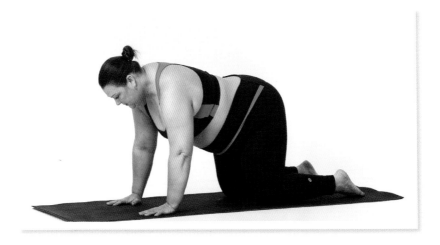

5. In Tabletop remember you can pad your knees with a blanket if they are tender.
6. Adjust your position so your elbows have a slight bend in them to protect your joints and you take some weight into your hands and fingers to protect the wrists before coming into Cat and Cow. (See pages 73–74 for Cat and Cow positions.)
7. Inhale and as you exhale drop your chin towards your chest and round your spine up towards the ceiling, drawing your navel in towards your spine.
8. As you inhale, lift your chin gently and lift your chest as you gently arch your spine (repeat 1–2 times).
9. Lower the front of your body onto the ground into Sphinx with your elbows roughly under your shoulders and your forearms and hands pointing forward. Lift a little through the chest and keep your chin parallel to the floor (take as many breaths here as you like, remember Crocodile is also a good option.) (See page 120.)
10. Inhale and as you exhale draw your hands back and lift your body up into Tabletop.

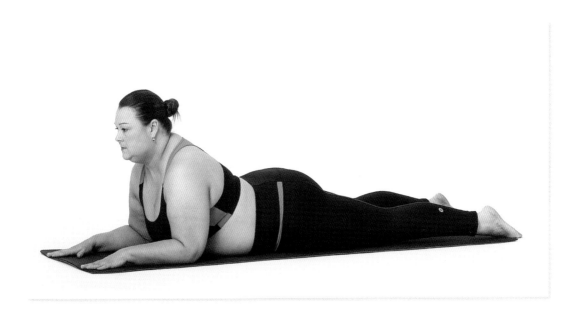

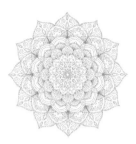

Widen your knees and sink your hips back towards your heels, stretching your arms out in front of you, shoulder width apart, with your head resting on the mat (or on two fists) in Child's Posture. Stay here for a few breaths (see pages 84–85 for Child's Posture). If Child's Posture isn't comfy for you, stay in Tabletop.

11. Come up to kneeling and bring the right leg forward, bent at the knee and tuck the toes of your left foot under. Focusing on your back leg, use that to lift your body off the ground and then draw it towards your left leg as you come to the standing forward bend, knees bent.

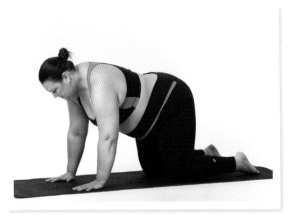

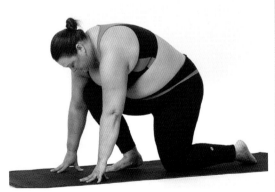

12. Very slowly come to standing, taking your arms wide and up over your head, palms together.

13. Slowly bring your hands together down the midline of your body to rest your thumbs on your heart in Prayer Position.

14. Repeat with the left leg leading and you have a complete round. Do as many rounds as you like!

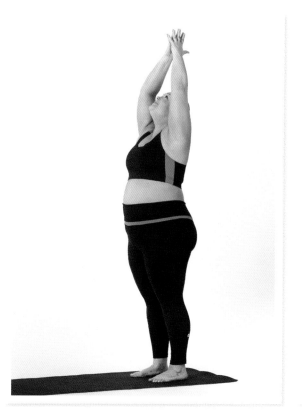

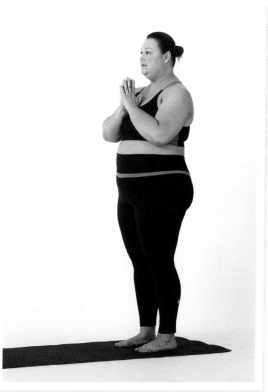

## SEATED POSTURES

### Hints and tips

» In most of the seated postures I would place a folded blanket under my hips to raise them and protect my joints.

» Some people find sitting cross-legged tough, so the Staff Posture (page 57) is a good substitute for a cross-legged position.

» All bodies look different in forward bends (sitting and standing) so be mindful that you can always pop a rolled up blanket under your knees to support them, and that touching your toes is only available to some people. Aim for a comfortable stretch instead.

» Make room for your individual body (belly and boobs!) by taking your legs a little wider anytime you like in seated or standing forward bends.

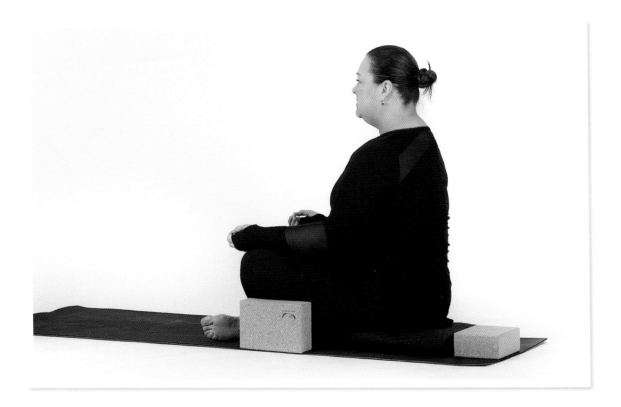

**Staff Posture – Dandasana**

1. Sit on the edge of a folded blanket with your legs straight out in front at hip width apart, toes pointing towards the ceiling, legs engaged.
2. Sit upright with a natural curve in your spine and relaxed shoulders.
3. Take your hands (or fingers) to the floor beside your hips.
4. Engage your legs and flex your feet back towards your face.
5. Breathe freely.

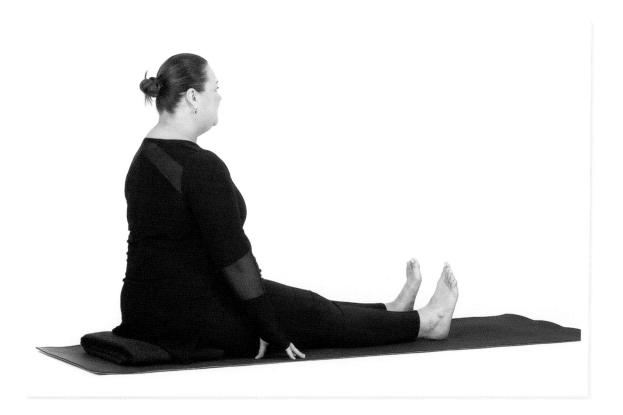

**Easy Posture – Sukhasana**

1. Sitting on the edge of a folded blanket, begin in Staff Posture (page 57) and cross your legs in the most comfortable position for you.
2. Sit upright, relax your shoulders and lift your chest slightly.
3. Bring your hands lightly to your knees.
4. If your knees are uncomfortable, return to Staff Posture or try placing blocks under each knee to support them.

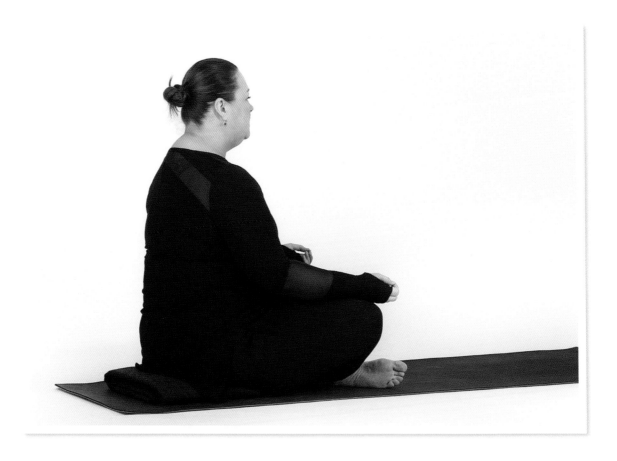

**Butterfly Posture – Baddha Konasana**

1. Sitting on the edge of a folded blanket, begin in Staff Posture (page 57) and bring the soles of your feet together in front of you.
2. The distance of your feet from your body is up to your individual body; I would encourage you to experiment with how far away is right for you.
3. Place your hands where they are comfortable on your knees or legs and either sit up tall or fold forward with your hands on the floor in front of you or on a bolster or block.
4. Breathe gently and stay in this posture for 5–10 breaths.

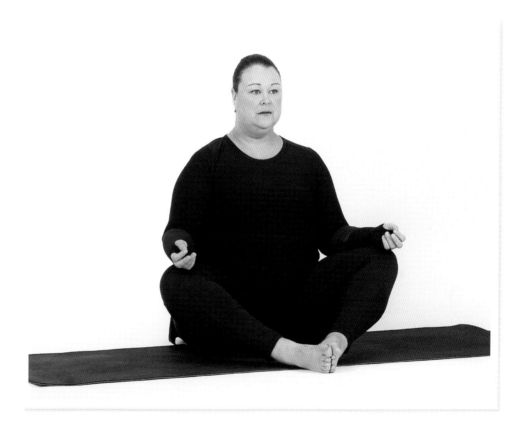

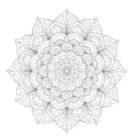

## Butterfly Posture version 2

1.  Add blocks under either knee to support a comfortable position for your knees and hips.

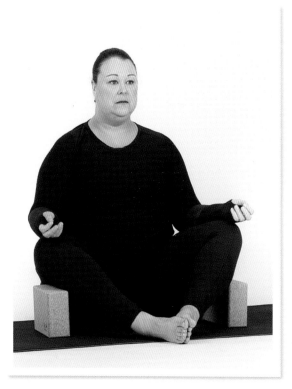 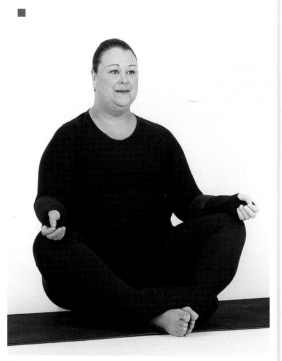

**Butterfly Posture version 3**

1.  Using your blanket, fold it on the longest edge in half and half again till it is a few inches wide.
2.  Place the front of the blanket over your feet and then take each edge and tuck the edges under each hip.
3.  The blanket should feel like a snug support for your body and not move around.
4.  Remain tall and breathe gently or fold forward from the hip joints and place your hands on the floor, or a block or bolster in front of you.

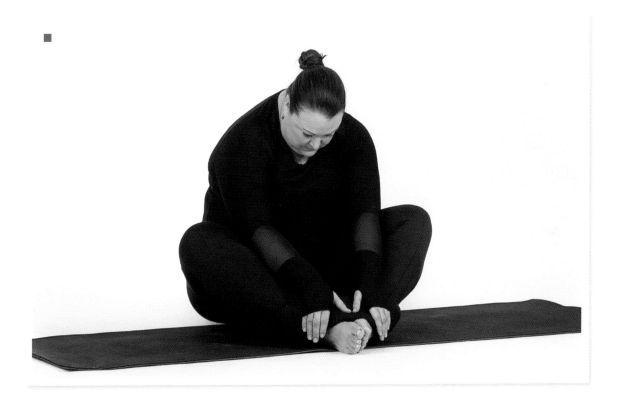

**Wide Leg Forward Bend – Upavistha Konasana**

1. Begin in Staff Posture (page 57) sitting on the edge of a folded blanket and take your legs our as wide as feels good to you, flexing your feet back towards your face.
2. With relaxed shoulders find the natural curve of your spine and inhale.
3. As you exhale fold forward from your hip joint, bringing your hands in front of you to the floor coming only as far forward as is comfortable (for some people this is not very far, with your hands on blocks, for others your forearms may be on the floor in front of you).
4. Stay here for 5–10 breaths before walking your hands back up, so your torso is in an upright position.

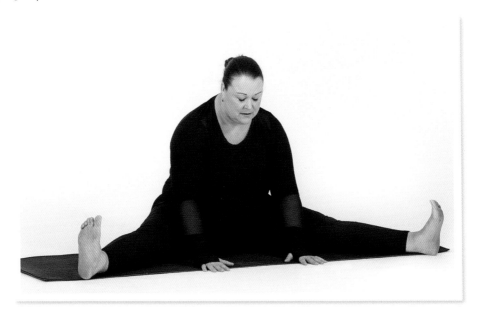

**Wide Leg Forward Bend version 2**

1. Using the bolster, position it lengthways in front of you and fold forward from your hips so that the short end of the bolster rests on your forehead.
2. Play around with the bolster and its position to find a really comfortable and supported forward bend.

**3.** Stay here for 5–10 breaths and slowly return to an upright position.

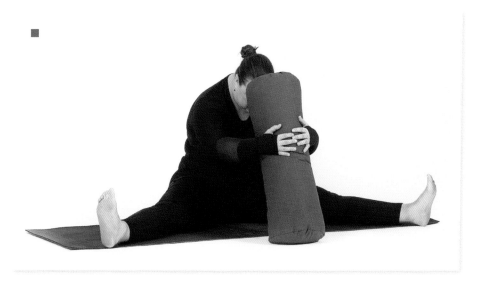

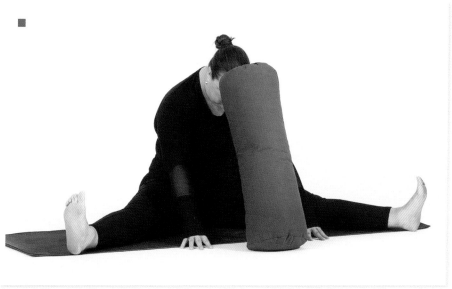

**Wide Leg Forward Bend version 3**

1.  Position your chair between your legs with the seat facing towards you and a folded blanket on the seat for support and comfort.
2.  Fold forward from your hips and bring your forearms to the seat of the chair and gently rest your forehead on your arms.
3.  Experiment with the distance of the chair from your body to find the most supportive forward bend for you.
4.  Stay here for 5–10 breaths.

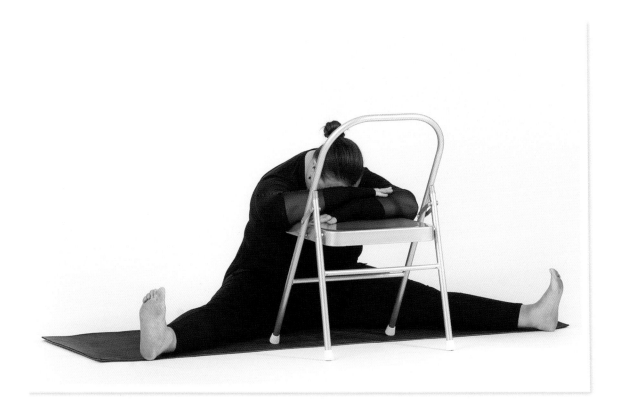

**Forward Bend – Paschimottanasana**

1.  Begin in Staff Posture (page 57) and on the inhale slowly raise your arms up overhead, relaxing your shoulders.
2.  On the exhale, draw in your abdominal muscles and slowly hinge forward from the hip joint bringing one hand to each side of the legs.
3.  Breathe here and with each exhale see if you can move a little further into the forward bend, keeping your shoulders relaxed and soft.
4.  Stay for 5–10 breaths.

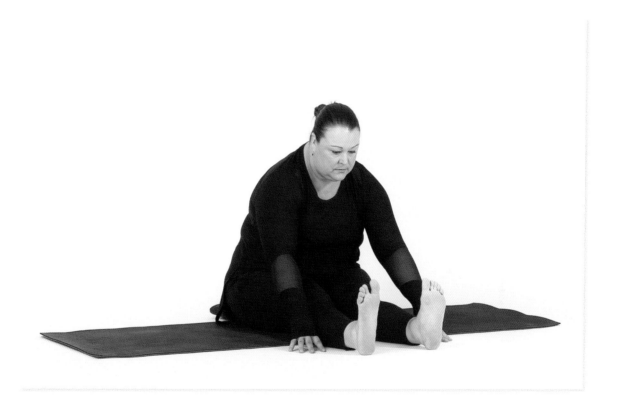

**Forward Bend version 2**

1. Begin in Staff Posture (page 57) with a rolled up blanket or bolster and strap nearby.
2. Take the rolled blanket/bolster and pop it under the back of your knees and then loop the strap around the balls of your feet.
3. Sitting up tall take one end of the strap in each hand, engage your abdominal muscles and on the exhale walk your hands down the strap towards your feet, hinging from your hips.
4. Stop at a comfortable point where you can breathe freely and your shoulders are relaxed. Stay here for 5–10 breaths and then slowly roll back up.

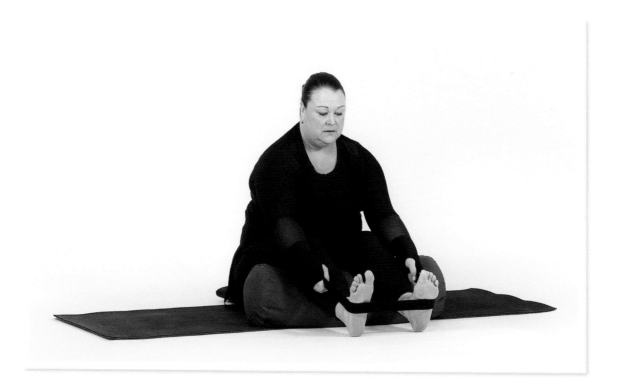

**Seated Cat – Marjariasana**

1. Sitting in the Staff Posture (page 57) bring your hands behind your neck, interlacing your fingers.
2. Engage your abdominals and inhale and as you exhale drop your chin towards your chest and draw your belly button towards your spine as you round your spine, bringing your elbows towards each other and rolling your shoulders forward.
3. Inhale and go straight into Seated Cow.

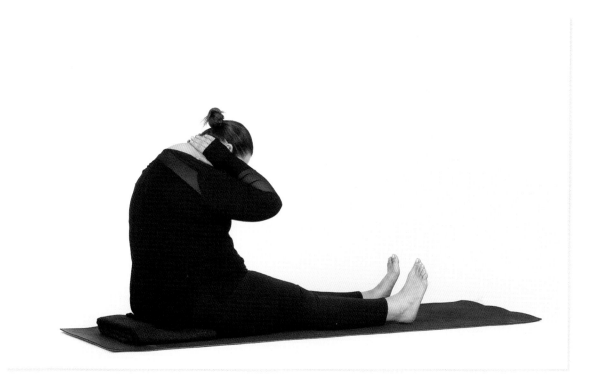

**Seated Cow – Bitilasana**

1. From Seated Cat, on the inhale keep your abdominals engaged and as you lift your chin and chest take your elbows back to shoulder height, drawing your shoulder blades together, gently arching through your spine.
2. Exhale and round your spine and roll your shoulders forward as you move back into the Seated Cat.
3. Do 2–5 rounds of the Cat and Cow combination.

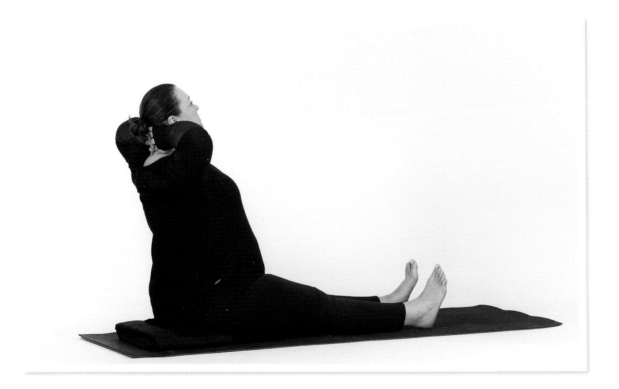

**Seated Twist – Matsyendrasana**

1. From Staff Posture (page 57) bend your right knee and place the sole of the foot on the floor, roughly in line with your hip, and take your right elbow and place it on the inner right knee.
2. Take your left hand to the floor behind you as you twist to the left, your head also moving to look over your left shoulder, if that suits your neck
3. If your left hand does not comfortably reach the floor, use a block underneath it (bringing the floor to you!).
4. Your chin is parallel to the floor and you lift your chest slightly, lightly pressing your elbow into your inner knee.
5. Stay here for 5–10 breaths and return your gaze forward first before untwisting and moving to the other side.

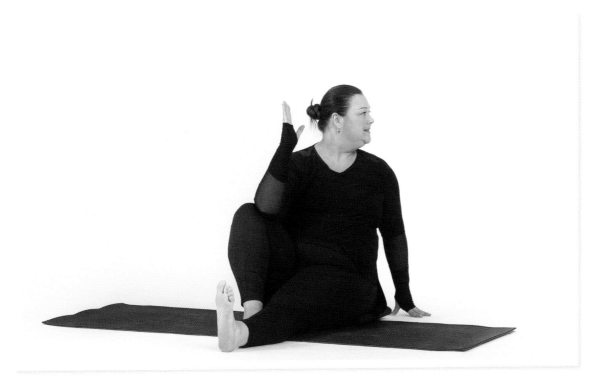

**Head to Knee Posture – Janu Sirsasana**

1. From the Staff Posture (page 57) bend your right leg and place the sole of the foot against the inside of the left thigh, where it is comfortable for the knee (if it's more like the foot is on the calf, then that is fine).
2. If either knee does not feel comfortable prop a block or blanket under the knee to support it.
3. Sit up with a natural curve in your spine and inhale your arms up overhead. As you exhale, fold forward from your hips, keeping your shoulders relaxed and your head looking down towards your leg.

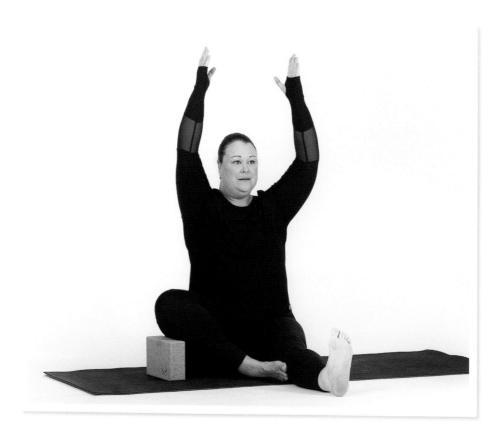

4. Your hands can come to either side of your left leg or rest on your body.
5. Although this is called 'head to knee' posture, there is no expectation that your head goes anywhere near your knee! (Mine doesn't!).
6. Stay here for 3–10 breaths.
7. Slowly bring your body to upright and draw your right leg back out in front of you to Staff Posture and repeat on the other side.

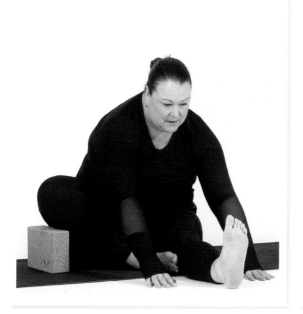
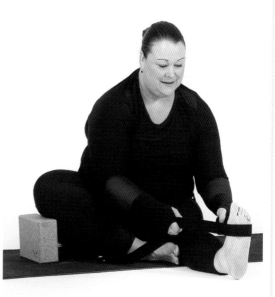

## KNEELING POSTURES

### Hints and Tips
» If your knees are tender then place a folded blanket underneath them.
» Many kneeling postures can be substituted for other postures, for example you can substitute the Cat and Cow with the Seated Cat and Cow on pages 67–68.

### Tabletop Position
1. Come onto your hands and knees, back firm and face parallel to the floor.
2. Your wrists should be roughly under your shoulders with your fingers pointing forward and a small bend in your elbows to protect your wrists.
3. Your knees should be under your hips with your feet in line with your knees.
4. Breathe freely and use this as the starting point for many of the kneeling positions.

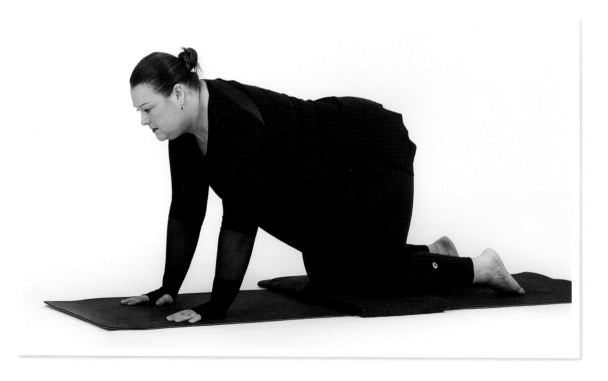

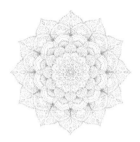

**Cat Posture – Marjariasana**

Note: linking Cat and Cow together can be a great quick warm-up!

1. From Tabletop Position, inhale and as you exhale begin to round your spine upwards towards the ceiling, drawing your abdominal muscles in towards your spine.
2. Move right into Cow Posture on the inhale.

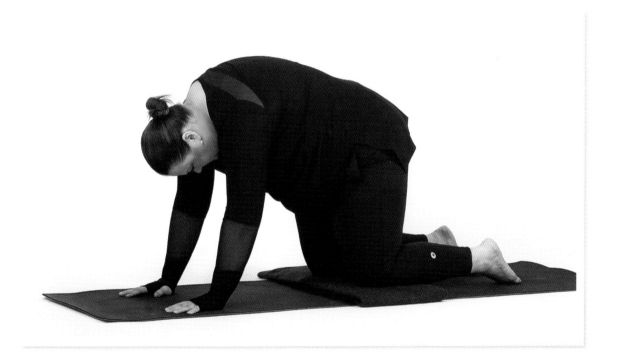

### Cow Posture – Bitilasana

1. From Cat Posture, inhale, and as you do lift your buttocks and chest slowly while lowering down the middle back as your chin comes up and your gaze is straight ahead (the spine is hollowed down as far as is comfortable).
2. Flowing with the breath (moving into Cat Posture on the exhale and Cow Posture on the inhale), continue through 5–10 rounds of Cat and Cow Postures linked together.

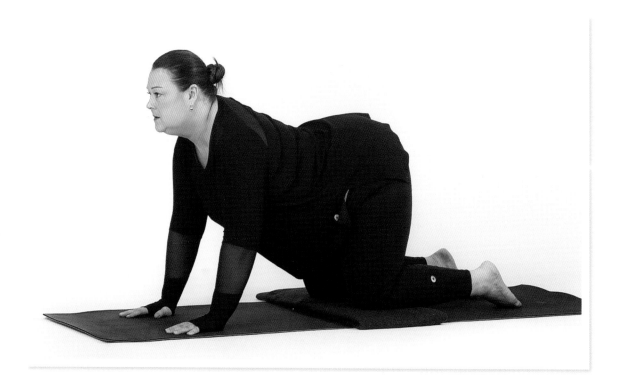

**Tiger Pose – Vyaghrasana**

1. From Tabletop (page 72) inhale and lift your right arm to shoulder height (palm facing in) and your left leg up to hip height.
2. Exhale and bring your arm and leg back down and repeat on the other side.
3. This is also a balance so if it feels more accessible (or even just as you build strength) you can just lift either your arm or your leg (work up to both!).

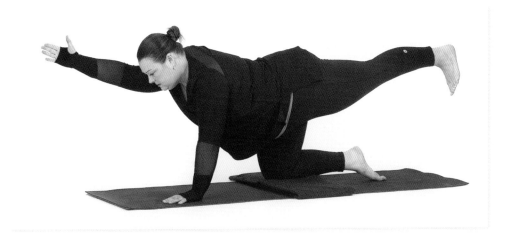

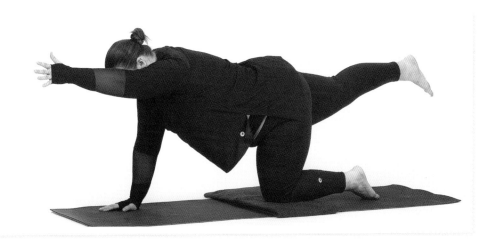

**Modified Wild Thing – Camatkarasana**

1. From Tabletop (page 72), take your right leg back behind your left heel (foot parallel to the short edge of the mat).
2. Move your left foot a few inches away from your body (outside the line of the knee) to create a stable base.
3. As you inhale, take your right hand off the floor and raise the arm above the head with your fingertips pointing towards the ceiling. Look towards your raised hand.
4. Stay here for a few breaths before bringing your hand down first and then drawing your leg back into Tabletop Position.
5. Repeat on the other side and a suggestion is to do 2–3 rounds.

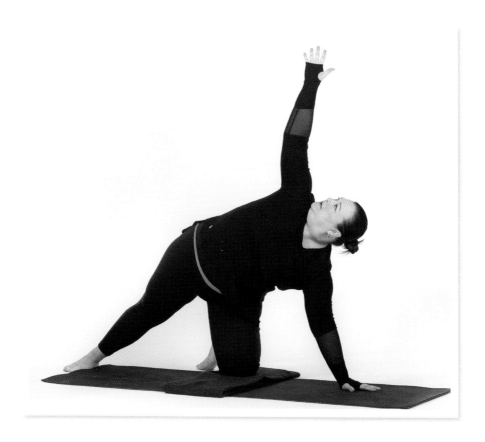

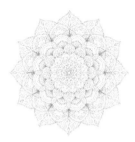

**Kneeling Position**

1.  From Tabletop (page 72), walk your hands back to come to a kneeling position.
2.  Your knees and feet are at hip distance apart.

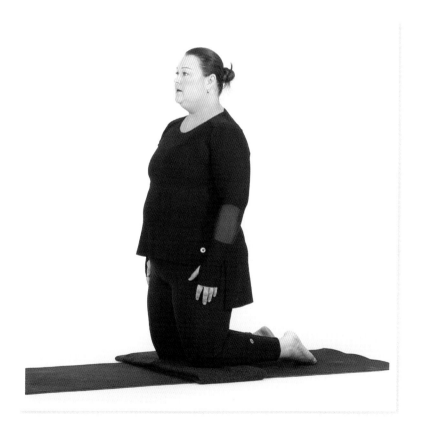

**Half Camel – Ardha Ustrasana**

1. Start in Kneeling Position (page 77). Find your bolster and place it on your lower calves.
2. Exhaling, take your right hand back behind you onto the bolster (near your right heel).
3. Inhale and take your left arm up towards the ceiling as you engage the front of your thighs and tuck your pelvis down slightly as you lift your chest and press your hips forward.
4. Take a few breaths here before exhaling your left hand down and returning to the Kneeling Position.
5. Repeat on the other side.
6. Tip for further practice: once you feel comfortable here you can try moving into the full Camel Position with both hands on the bolster!

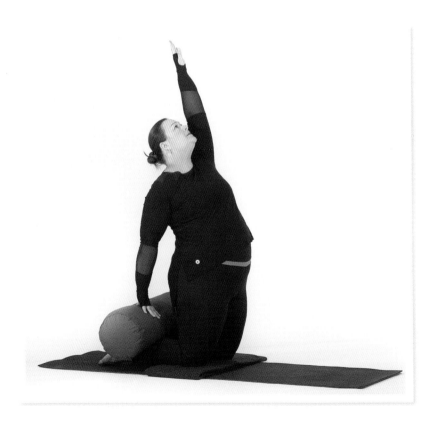

**Low Lunge – Anjaneyasana**

1. From the Kneeling Position (page 77), step your right foot forward towards the front of your mat.
2. Sink your hips forward into the lunge being careful that your right knee doesn't travel beyond your right ankle.
3. Your hands can stay at your heart in Prayer Position or you can inhale them up and over your head, looking up.
4. Stay here for 5 breaths and exhale your arms down, pressing though your right foot to bring your hips back to above your left knee and come back to kneeling before moving to the other side.

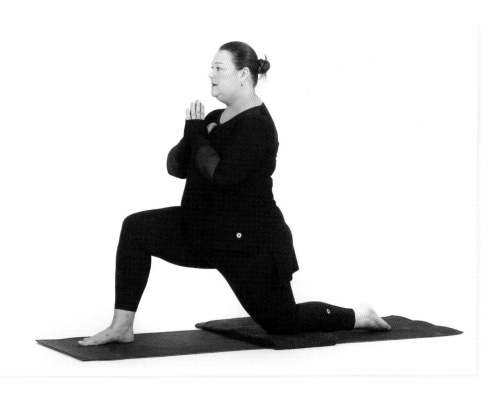

## Low Lunge version 2

1. Start in the Kneeling Position (page 77), find your bolster and place it under your left knee and shin and step forward with your right foot.
2. Sink your hips forward into the lunge with your right knee positioned over your right ankle.
3. Your hands can stay at your heart in Prayer Position or you can inhale them up and over your head, looking up.
4. Stay here for 5 breaths and exhale your arms down, pressing though your right foot to bring your hips back to above your left hip and come back to kneeling before moving to the other side.

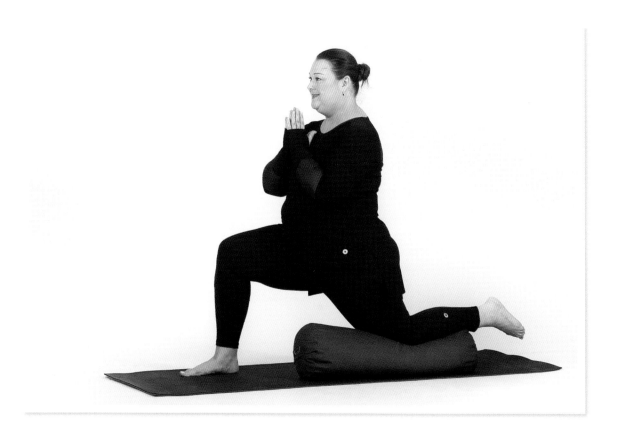

**Pigeon – Eka Pada Rajakapotasana**

Note: Pigeon is a posture people can find uncomfortable! If it hurts your knees or isn't right for your body, then come to version 3, the lovely lying Pigeon!

1. From Tabletop (page 72) come into Downward Facing Dog (page 126).
2. Draw your right knee in behind your right wrist while sinking your torso to the mat taking your left leg straight behind you. Your right foot is pointing towards your left knee.
3. Take a rolled up blanket and place under your right hip for joint and pelvic support.
4. Keeping your hands on the floor or bolster, stay here for 5–10 breaths before tucking your left toes under and drawing your right leg back into Downward Facing Dog.
5. Repeat on the other side.

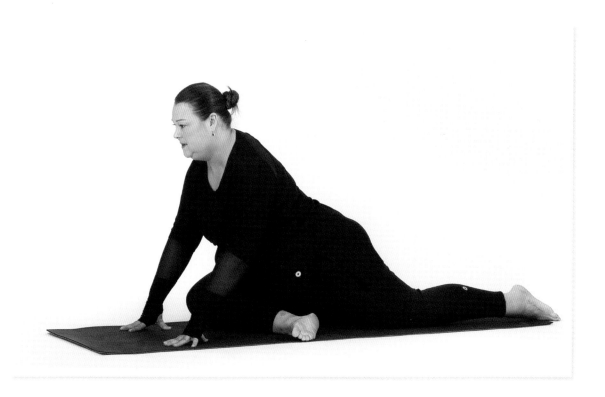

**Pigeon version 2**

1. Begin in Kneeling Position (page 77) with a bolster across the front of your mat.
2. Step your right foot over the bolster and walk or move the right foot in front of the left knee.
3. With your hands on the bolster take the left leg back behind you.
4. You can keep your torso upright and your hands on the bolster or fold forward with your hands on the floor in front of you.
5. Stay here for 5–10 breaths then return to upright, tuck your back toes under and bring your right leg back to high kneeling, untuck the toes and move to the other side.

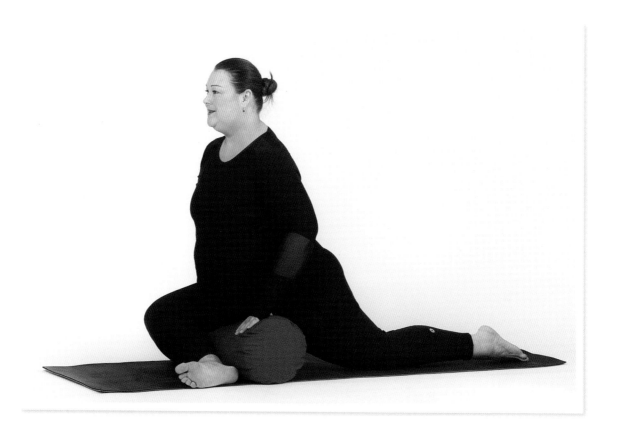

**Pigeon version 3**

1. Place a bolster across the front of your mat.
2. Lie on your back with your knees bent up and your arms relaxed by your body.
3. Take your right foot off the floor and place your right ankle on your left knee and your right knee will fall out to the side. Flex your right foot to protect the knee joint.
4. Lift your left foot off the floor and place it on the bolster.
5. Find a comfortable point and hold for 5–10 breaths before moving to the other side.

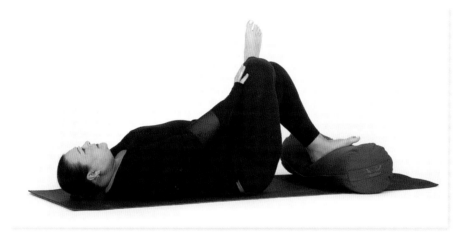

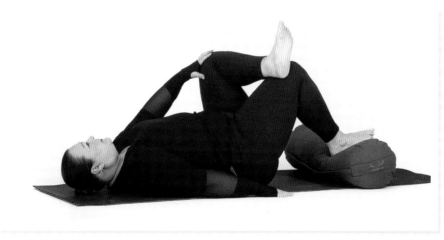

### Extended Child's Posture – Balasana

Note: not everyone feels comfy in Child's Posture and if that's the case for you just stay in Tabletop (page 72) or Cat/Cow (pages 73–74)) if you are in a studio class, or try the restorative version on (page 135).

1. From Tabletop (page 72) take your knees wide with your toes pointing towards each other.
2. Sink your hips back towards your heels (they don't need to be close!) as you make two fists with your hands in front of you and rest your forehead on your fists.
3. Stay here for 5–10 breaths.

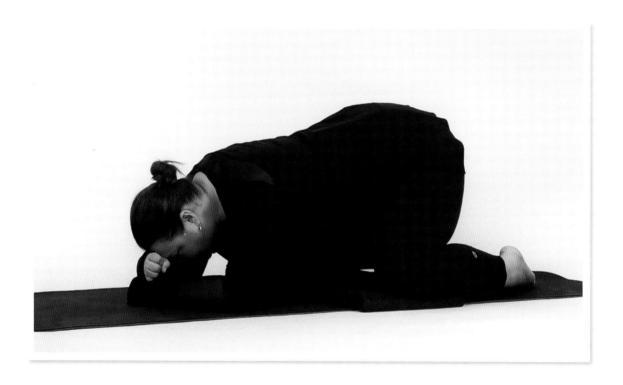

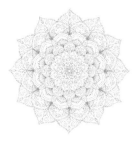

## Extended Child's Posture version 2

1.  From Tabletop, widen your knees a little with your toes pointing towards each other.
2.  Keeping your hands on the floor in front of you just sink your hips a little towards your heels, stopping when you feel comfortable.
3.  Stay here for 5–10 breaths.

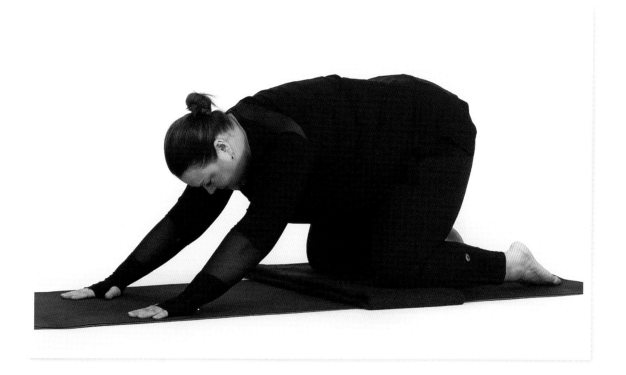

## STANDING POSTURES

### Mountain Posture – Tadasana

1. Stand with your feet hip distance apart, a micro-bend in your knees, lifting up through the arches of your feet.
2. Draw your shoulder blades down slightly and lift your chest, engaging your abdominals.
3. Hands and arms are relaxed beside you.
4. Your chin is parallel to the floor, close your eyes if you feel balanced.
5. Stay here, feeling into the whole body, for 5–10 breaths.

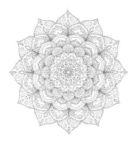

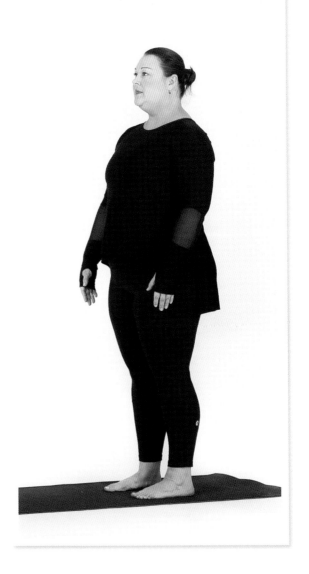

### Triangle – Trikonasana

1. Stand towards the back of your mat in Mountain Posture (page 86).
2. Inhale as you step your right foot forward, keeping hips squared towards the front of the mat.
3. Exhale and take your arms in front of you at shoulder height, palms together.
4. Inhale and extend your arms forward from the hips to a comfortable point.
5. Exhale and bring your right hand to the inside of the right ankle (or knee or block).
6. Inhale as you take your left hand towards the ceiling, looking up, leaving your right hand on the block or inner leg, twisting through the hips.
7. Stay here for 3–8 breaths then bring the left hand down to meet the right, palms touching, bend the right knee deeply as you bring your torso up (engaging your abdominals) and your arms to shoulder height.
8. Drop your arms down beside you and step forward.
9. Return to the back of your mat in Mountain Posture and repeat on the other side.

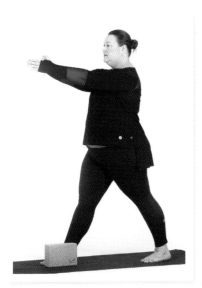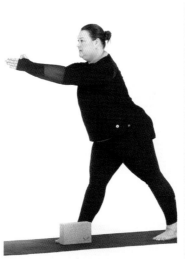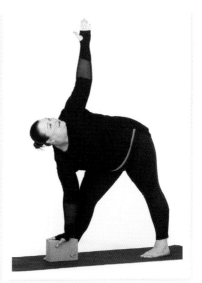

**Triangle version 2**

1. Place a chair in front of you (seat facing towards you), about a meter away.
2. Begin in Mountain Posture (page 86) and step your right foot forward (it should land just on the inside of the front right leg of the chair) and bend the knee slightly.
3. Inhale and take your arms up to shoulder height in front of you with your palms together.
4. Exhale and take both hands to the seat of the chair.
5. Inhale take the left hand towards the ceiling, looking up, twisting through the hips, your right hand roughly under your right shoulder.
6. Stay here for 3–8 breaths before bringing your left arm down to the chair, bending your right leg and stepping the left leg forward and then slowly rolling up to standing.
7. Step back to the original position before repeating on the other side.

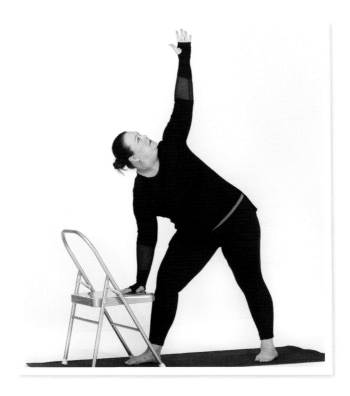

### Pyramid Posture – Parsvottanasana

1. From Mountain Posture (page 86) step your right foot forward, squaring your hips towards the front of the mat (if you want to make a more stable base walk your right foot out to the right slightly).
2. Bend your right knee so it is over your ankle.
3. Inhale and lift your arms above your head, relaxing your shoulders, chin parallel to the floor.
4. Exhale as you fold forward, bringing your torso toward your right thigh and one hand on either side of your right foot, straightening your right leg, but not locking the knee.
5. Relax your head and neck and breathe here, taking even weight between your front and back foot.
6. Stay here for 3–8 breaths before inhaling and bending your right knee deeply, engaging your abdominal muscles and sweeping your arms back above your head.
7. Exhale and bring your arms back down, straighten your front leg and step forward, back to Mountain Posture. Repeat on the opposite side.

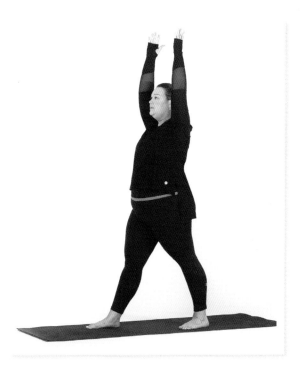

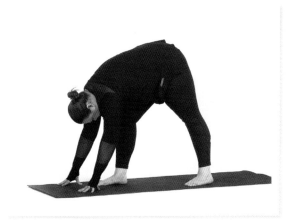

**Pyramid Posture version 2**

1. Position a chair in front of you (seat facing towards you), about a meter away.
2. From Mountain Posture (page 86) step your right foot forward, squaring your hips towards the front of the mat (if you want to make a more stable base walk your right foot out to the right slightly).
3. Bend your right knee so it is over your ankle.
4. Inhale and lift your arms above your head, relaxing your shoulders, chin parallel to the floor.
5. Exhale and fold forward, bringing your forearms to the seat or top of the chair, relaxing your head.
6. Stay here for 3–8 breaths before inhaling and bending your right knee deeply, engaging your abdominal muscles and sweeping your arms back above your head.
7. Exhale and bring your arms back down, straighten your front leg and step forward, back to Mountain Posture. Repeat on the opposite side.

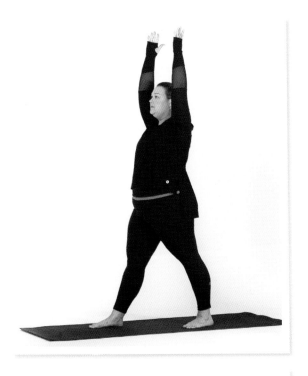

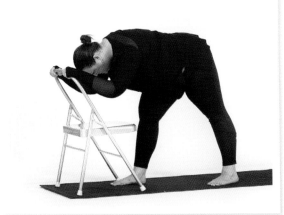

**Warrior 1 – Virabhadrasana 1**

1. From Mountain Posture (page 86) step your right foot forward, squaring your hips towards the front of the mat (if you want to make a more stable base walk your front foot out to the right slightly).
2. Bend your right knee so it is over your ankle.
3. Inhale and slowly lift your arms above your head (drawing your arm bones into the sockets) relaxing your shoulders, chin parallel to the floor. Breathe freely.
4. Press down evenly into the back and front foot and lift your chest slightly, feeling strong and warrior-like!
5. Stay here for 3–8 breaths and either flow into Warrior 2 or on the exhale bring your arms down beside you, deepen your knee bend and step forwards to Mountain Posture.
6. Come to the back of your mat to repeat on the other side.

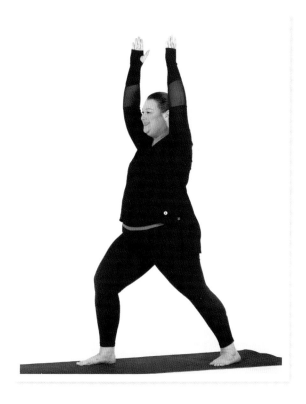

**Warrior 2**

1. From Warrior 1, with the right leg forward, drop your right arm in front of you at shoulder height as you bring the back arm behind you at shoulder height.
2. Let your torso and hips naturally open up to the left at the same time.
3. Pivot on your back foot so it's parallel to the short edge of the mat.
4. Your gaze is down the front middle finger. Press evenly into both feet, lifting your chest and keeping your torso in the midline.
5. Breathe here for 3–8 breaths before bringing your arms down pivoting onto your toes on the back foot and turning your hips so they are square to the front of the mat.
6. Bend your front knee and press off through the back foot, stepping forward into Mountain Posture.
7. Repeat on the other side.

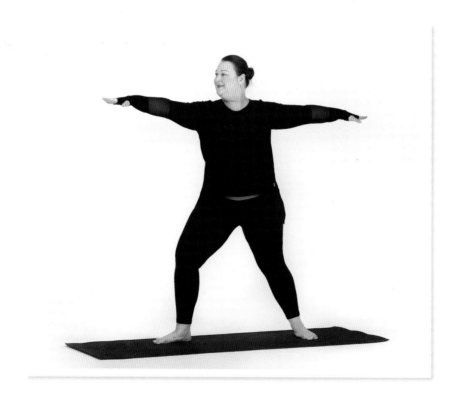

**Warrior 3**

1. Begin in Mountain Posture (page 86) standing about a leg's length away from a wall (facing out).
2. Take your right leg back behind you so your foot finds the wall and can comfortably press into it for support.
3. Square your hips towards the ground, find your balance and lift your arms up in front of you at shoulder height with your gaze down towards the floor.
4. Breathe here for 3–8 breaths before activating your abdominal muscles to bring your right foot back to the floor and repeating on the other side.

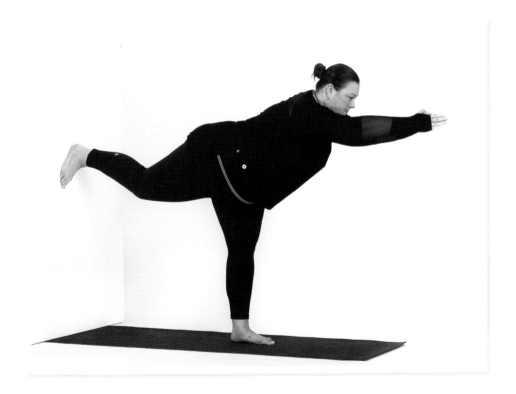

**Warrior 3 version 2**

1. Begin in Mountain Posture with a chair in front of you, seat facing away from you. Bend your knees softly and fold forward from your hips bringing your hands or forearms to the top of the chair back.
2. From here, if you feel steady, raise your right leg up behind you as far as is comfortable (around hip height), flexing your foot and gazing down so your neck is long.
3. Stay here for 3–5 breaths before bending your left knee, engaging your stomach muscles and bringing your right foot to the floor.
4. Repeat on the other side.

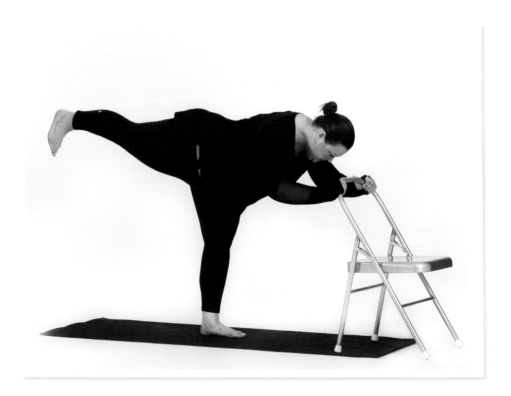

**Wide Leg Forward Bend – Prasarita Padottanasana**

1. Place your blocks in the middle of your mat. From Mountain Posture (page 86) at the top of your mat, turn to face the long edge of the mat, bend your knees and step your left foot out as far as you comfortably can, turning your toes in slightly.
2. Bending forward from your hips, fold forward so your hands are on your blocks or your forearms are resting on your knees.
3. Relax your head and shoulders and breathe here for 3–7 breaths then bend your knees deeply and, using your stomach muscles, return to standing.
4. Repeat, or walk or step your feet back together.

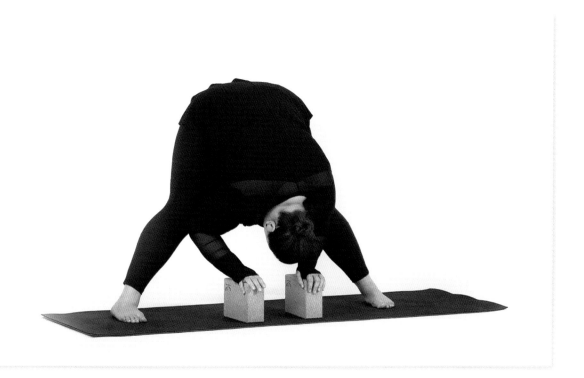

**Wide Leg Forward Bend version 2**

1.  Place your chair in the middle of your mat with the seat facing towards you
2.  From Mountain Posture (page 86) at the top of your mat, turn to face the long edge of the mat, bend your knees and step your left foot out as far as you comfortably can, turning your toes in slightly.
3.  Bending forward from your hips, fold forward so your hands and forearms are resting on the seat of the chair.
4.  Relax your head and shoulders and breathe here for 3–7 breaths, bend your knees deeply and using your stomach muscles return to standing.
5.  Repeat, or walk or step your feet back together.

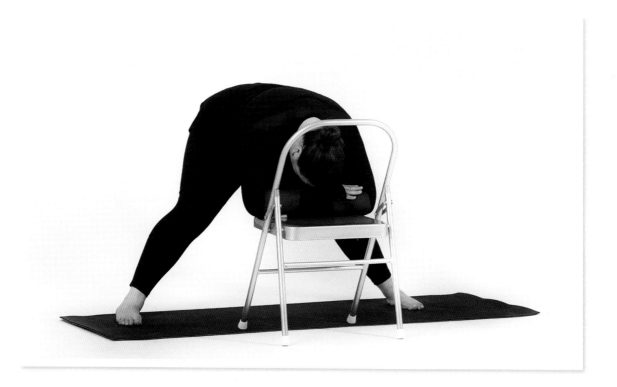

## Chair Pose – Utkatasana

1. Begin in Mountain Posture (page 86), inhale and take your arms up overhead, relax your face and shoulders.
2. Exhale and sink your hips like you are going to sit on a chair and bend your knees (knees are over feet).
3. Breathing freely, engage your abdominal muscles and legs.
4. Stay here for 3–8 breaths before bringing your arms back down beside you and straightening your legs.
5. Repeat if you like!

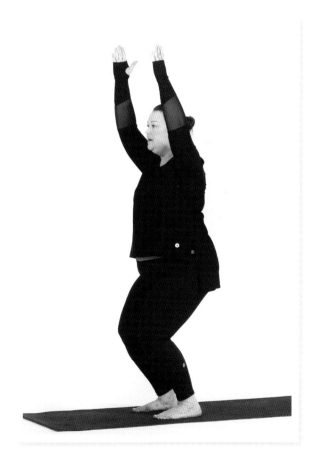

**Chair Pose version 2**

1. Begin in Mountain Posture (page 86) against a wall, your bottom should be resting lightly on the wall.
2. Inhale and take your arms up overhead, relax your face and shoulders.
3. Exhale and sink your hips like you are going to sit on a chair and bend your knees (knees are over feet), your back should rest lightly on the wall for as much support as you need.
4. Breathing freely, engage your abdominal muscles and legs.
5. Stay here for 3–8 breaths before bringing your arms back down beside you and straightening your legs.
6. Repeat if you like!

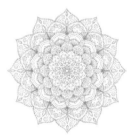

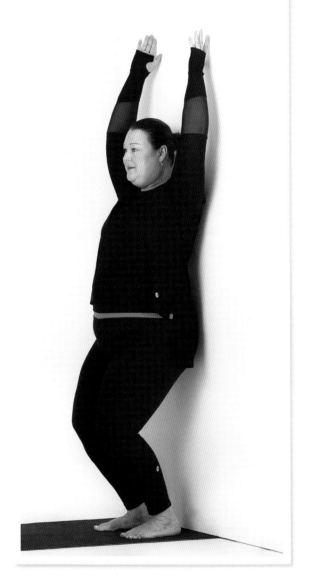

## Swan dive forward bend

1. Begin in Mountain Posture (page 86) and inhale as you take your arms out to the side with your palms facing up and you take your arms all the way overhead so your palms connect. Look up if it suits your neck.

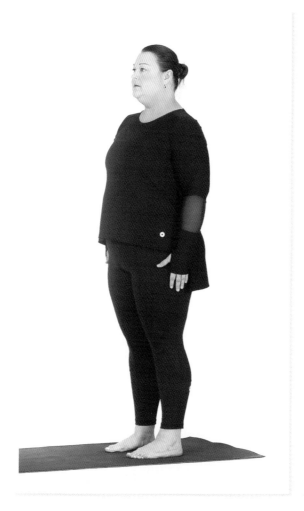
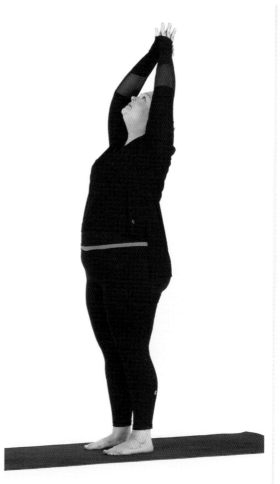

**2.** Exhale and separate your hands out to the side (palms facing away from you) as you lead with your chest and fold forward from your hips, bringing your forearms to rest on your knees, taking your feet a little wider if you need to.

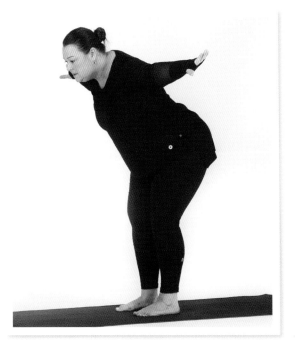

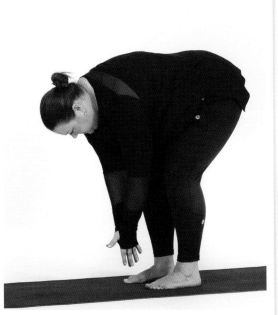

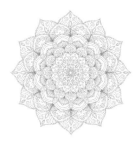

3. Inhale as you engage your abdominals, bend a little more in the knees and sweep your arms out to the side (palms facing away from you), lifting and expanding your chest as you bring your arms back up above your head, palms together.
4. Flow through this forward bend 3–5 times.

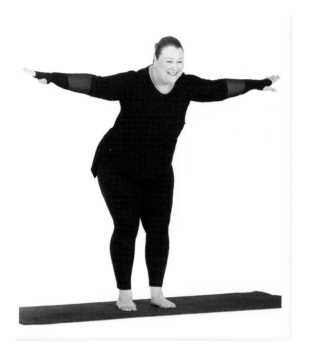 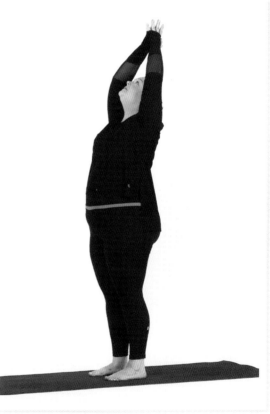

## BALANCE POSTURES

### Basic Balance

1. Begin in Mountain Posture (page 86), inhale and take your right foot in front of your left foot, with a little bend in your knees, and balance here.
2. If you would like to increase the balance, close your eyes.
3. Breathe freely for 3–8 breaths before taking your right foot back into Mountain Posture and then moving to the other side.

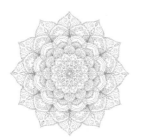

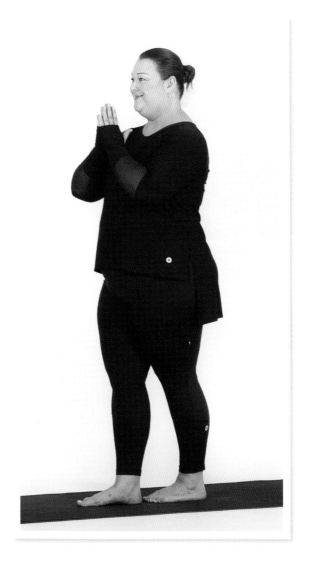

**Tree Posture – Vriksasana**

1. Begin in Mountain Posture (page 86), lift your right foot and place your right heel on your left ankle, rotating your knee and hip out to the side.
2. Engage your abdominals, have a small bend in the left leg and lift your heart center, bringing your hands into Prayer Position in front of your heart.
3. Either stay here or lift your right foot onto your calf and take your arms up overhead, your gaze is straight ahead.
4. Breathe here for 5–10 breaths before returning your foot to the floor and moving to the other side.

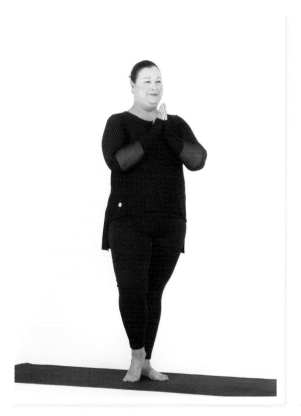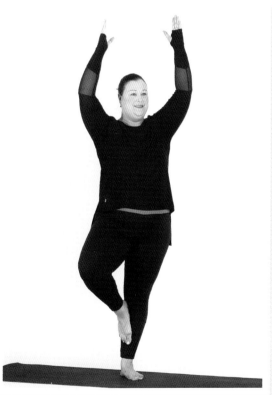

**Eagle Posture – Garudasana**

1. Place a block beside your left foot and begin in Mountain Posture (page 86), bend your left knee slightly and take your right leg over your left knee and either tuck it behind the left calf or onto the block.

2. Cross your left elbow above your right elbow and bring your left hand around to take your right hand (wrists cross), your forearms will be just in front of your face, gaze is forward.

3. Breathe freely here for 3–5 breaths before unhooking the arms and legs, coming back to Mountain Posture and repeating on the other side (this time crossing your right elbow above your left).

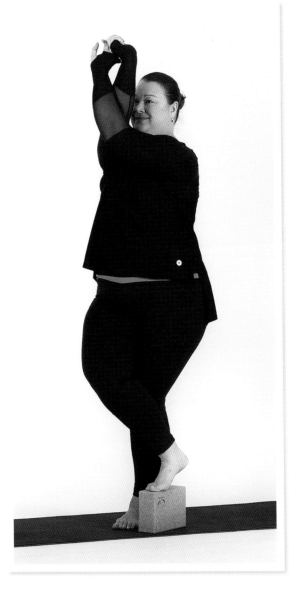

**Eagle Posture version 2**

1. Place a block beside your left foot and begin in Mountain Posture (page 86), bend your left knee slightly and take your right leg over your left knee and either tuck it behind the left calf or onto the block.

2. Wrap your arms around you by bringing one hand to the outside of each shoulder, crossing your left elbow above your right (elbows will be about chin height).

3. Breathe freely here for 3–5 breaths before unhooking the arms and legs, coming back to Mountain Posture and repeating on the other side (this time crossing your right elbow above your left).

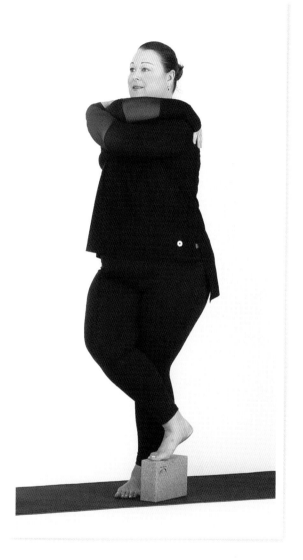

## Half Moon Posture – Ardha Chandrasana

1. Come to the Mountain Posture (page 86) with your back a couple of inches away from the wall.

2. Place a block near your left foot (which is parallel to the wall) and angle your right foot out slightly.

3. As you engage your abdominal muscles use the wall as support as you reach your left hand down to block and lift your right leg up to hip height and your right hand up and over your shoulder.

4. The back of your body can be partially supported by the wall as you lift up and out of your hips rotating them forward.

5. Only stay here as long as you feel stable and supported.

6. Come out of this pose carefully, using your leg and abdominal strength in preference to your back to lift your left arm as you bring your leg to the floor and the right arm down beside you.

7. Move your block to right side and repeat on the other side.

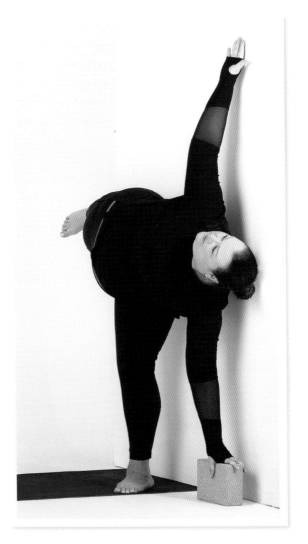

### Boat Posture flowing – Navasana

1. Come to a seated position at the front of your mat with both your knees bent up at the edge of your mat so your feet are on the floor (this needs to be a smooth, hard surface to work!) on a folded blanket.

2. Inhale and bring your arms up to shoulder height in front of you, palms facing in, and engage your abdominal muscles as you lean back slightly. Exhale.

3. As you inhale gently push your feet on the blanket away from you till your knees are almost flat and then exhale and slide them back towards you till your knees are bent up again.

4. Repeat as many times as you like before bringing your arms back down and sitting up straight in Easy Posture (page 58) or Staff Posture (page 57).

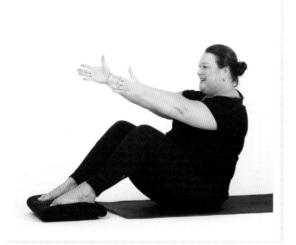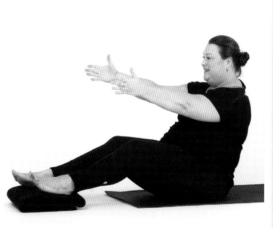

## SUPINE POSTURES: ON BACK

### Bridge Posture – Setu Bandhasana

1. Begin lying on your back with your knees bent up, about hip width apart, soles of the feet on the floor.
2. On the inhale, take your arms up and over your head slowly (they may not reach the floor, remember your own range of movement!).
3. On the exhale, slowly bring them back down beside you.
4. Repeat 2–5 time times with your breath.
5. Depending on your energy you can flow on to the next pose from here.

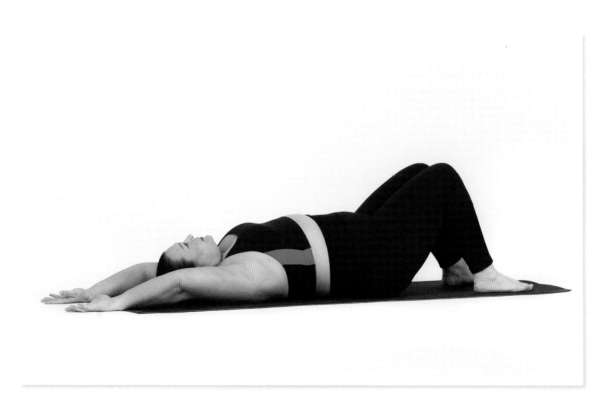

**Bridge Posture version 2**

1. Begin lying on your back with your knees bent up.
2. You may like to walk your feet a little back towards your buttocks and make sure your knees are hip width apart.
3. On the inhale lift your arms up and over your head as you press down into your feet and lift your hips and pelvis as high as is comfortable.
4. On the exhale, slowly bring your hips and spine back to the ground and your arms back down beside you.
5. Repeat 2–5 times and you might like to hold one of the lifts (don't forget to breathe), but it's up to you.

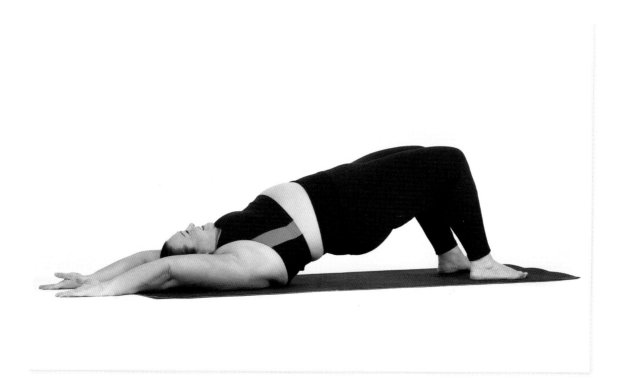

**Bridge Posture version 3**

1. Begin lying on your back with your knees bent up with a block nearby.
2. You may like to walk your feet a little back towards your buttocks and make sure your knees are hip width apart.
3. On the inhale press down into your feet and lift your hips and pelvis as high as is comfortable as you take the block and place it under your pelvis (not on your spine).
4. Relax your body and take your arms out to the side, palms down.
5. This is a restorative posture so you are welcome to stay here for 2–7 minutes with your eyes closed, just relaxing and focusing on your breath.
6. When you are ready, reach down and lift your hips slightly to take the block out and gently return your hips and spine to the ground.
7. Allow yourself a few moments (or more) to enjoy the effects of this posture! (I find it delicious!).

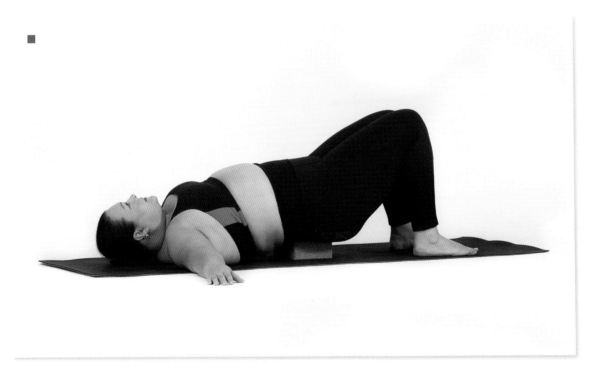

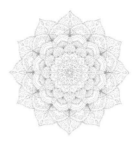

**Lying Twist – Supta Matsyendrasana**

1. Lie on your back with your knees bent up.
2. Inhale as you engage your core and lift your feet off the floor and bring your heels in line with your knees.
3. Exhale and take your arms out to shoulder height.
4. Inhale bring your knees and feet as close together as you can.

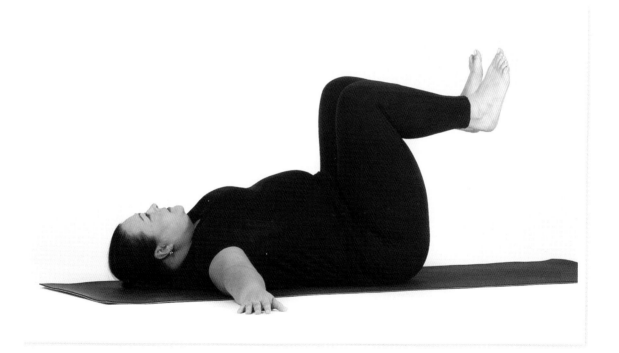

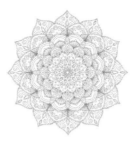

5. Exhale and carefully take your knees towards the floor on the right, keeping them stacked if that is comfortable, or moving them slightly apart if you like.
6. Your gaze can be turning toward your knees, looking up or away to the left (whatever is comfy for your neck).
7. Breathe here for 5–10 breaths or for a long hold if you like.
8. Activate your abdominal muscles to bring both knees back to center before dropping them to the left side and repeating.

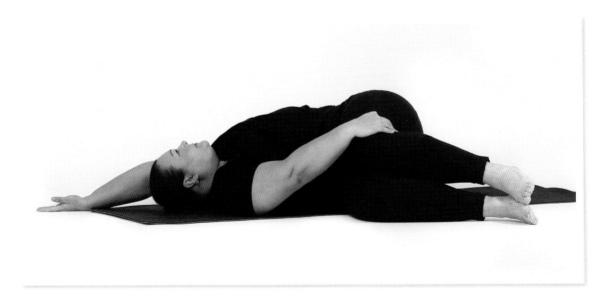

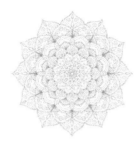

## Lying Twist version 2

1. Lie on your back with your knees bent and feet flat on the floor.
2. Inhale and take your arms out to shoulder height.
3. Exhale and walk your feet as wide as the mat.
4. Inhale and as you exhale drop your knees over to the right, making any adjustments (or even placing a blanket under the right knee to support it if you need to).

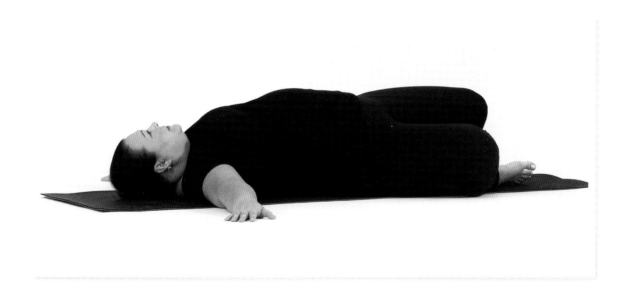

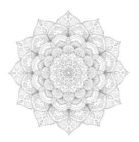

5. Breathe here for 5–10 breaths or for a long hold if you like.
6. Activate your abdominal muscles to bring both knees back to center before dropping them to the left side and repeating.

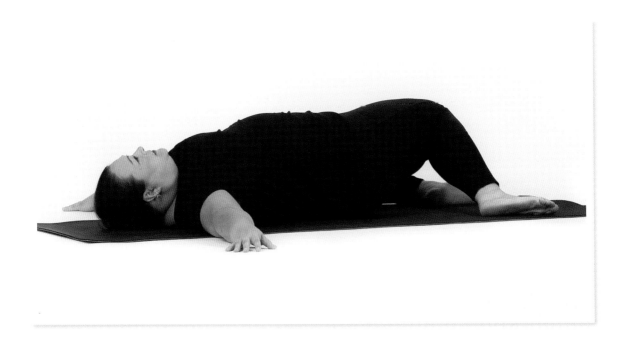

**Knees to Chest – Pawanmuktasana**

1. I have offered three versions of this position, as sometimes people don't find it comfortable with boobs and bellies in the way!
2. Lie on your back and bend your knees in towards your chest.
3. Take your knees wider than hip distance to make room for your body and so you can breathe freely.
4. Wrap your arms around your knees and relax your head and neck.
5. Breathe gently here (sometimes rocking gently from side to side is nice) for 5–10 breaths.

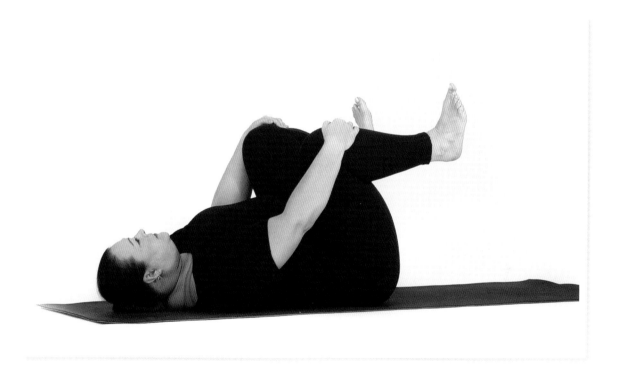

**Knees to Chest version 2**

In this version we will utilize the strap so place that in your most comfortable hand as you come to lying.

1.  Bring the strap behind your knees, walking your hands as close as they need to be so you are comfy and your body doesn't feel squished!
2.  Take your knees wide (up to you how wide, you can experiment with what feels comfortable) and relax your head and neck towards the floor.
3.  Breathe gently here (sometimes rocking gently from side to side is nice) for 5–10 breaths.

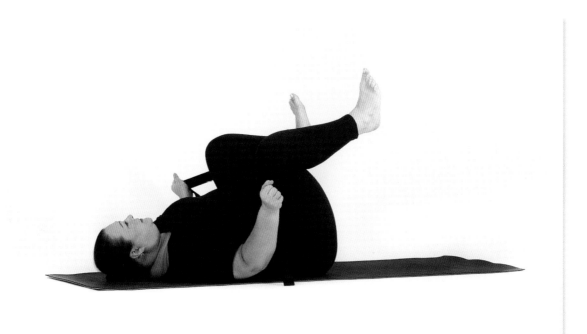

**Knees to Chest version 3**

1.  Lie on your back and in this version just bend your right leg in towards your chest, leaving the left leg bent with the foot on the floor.
2.  Your right hand can be on the knee, behind it, or you can use a strap.
3.  Relax your head and neck towards the floor.
4.  Breathe gently here (sometimes rocking gently from side to side is nice) for 5–10 breaths.

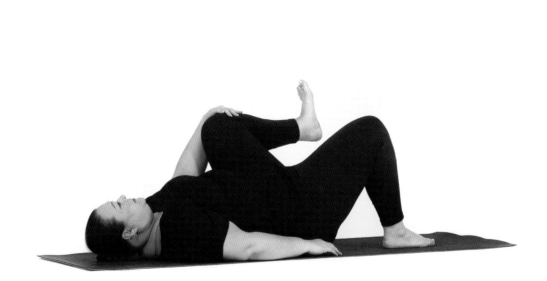

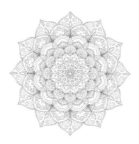

## Posture of Surrender – Savasana

This is often the final posture in a traditional practice.

1. Lie on your back with your legs straight out in front of you, hip width apart, feet falling gently out to the side. Arms should be a comfortable distance away from your body, palms facing up and hands relaxed.
2. Breathe in and out through your nose and close your eyes, if this suits you.
3. Stay here in stillness (in silence, or with relaxing music or my Savasana script on page 142) for 7–10 minute or longer, making sure to cover yourself if you are cool.

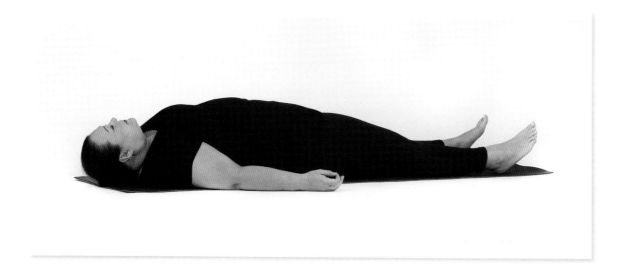

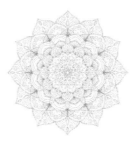

**Posture of Surrender version 2**

This is my favorite version of Savasana.

1. Lie on your back and place your bolster under your knees with your feet a little wider than hip width apart and feet falling open softly. Arms should be a comfortable distance away from your body, palms facing up and hands relaxed.

2. Place a blanket under your neck for support and use an eye bag if you like them. Cover yourself with a blanket if it's cool.

3. Breathe in and out through your nose and close your eyes, if this suits you.

4. Stay here in stillness (in silence or with relaxing music or my Savasana script on page 142) for 7–10 minute or longer.

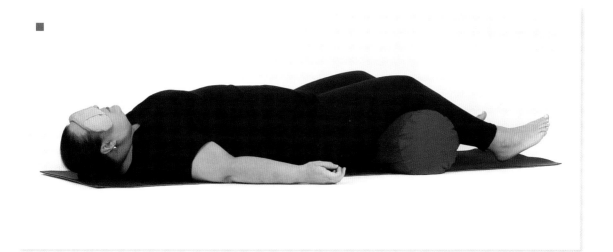

## PRONE POSTURES: ON FRONT

### Crocodile Posture – Makarasana

1. Lie on your front with your legs a little more than hip distance apart.
2. Bring your arms in front of you and raise your head and chest off the mat.
3. Take your right elbow or forearm with the left hand and the left elbow or forearm with your right hand.
4. Your gaze is looking just in front of your arms so your neck is long.
5. Close your eyes and relax your whole body.
6. Stay here for 5–10 breaths or a longer hold if you prefer.

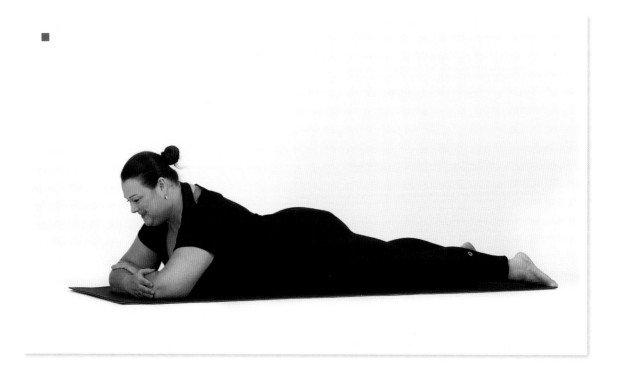

**Locust Posture – Salabhasana**

1. Lie on your front with your arms out in front of you on the floor and your legs at hip width apart, tuck the pelvis under slightly to protect the lower back.

2. Inhale and bring your arms back behind you, exhale and then on the next inhale lift your arms and front body off the mat, palms facing inward, using your abdominal muscles to stabilize you.

3. Take a few breaths here, before bringing your arms in front of you and relaxing your whole body onto the floor, head on your hands.

4. Return to the original position with your arms on the floor behind you and this time inhale and take your arms, chest and legs off the mat, using your abdominals and lower back to stabilize you.

5. Breathe here for 3–5 breaths before returning your legs and arms to the floor and bringing your arms in front of you resting your head on your hands and completely let go and relax, breathing gently.

6. Repeat if you like!

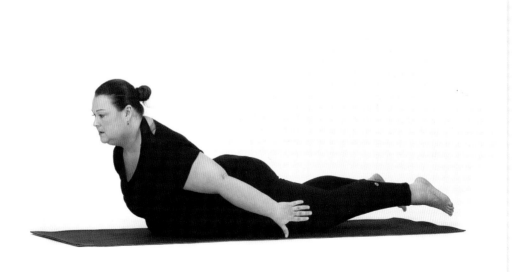

**Locust Posture version 2**

1. Lie on your front with two blocks nearby and legs hip distance apart.
2. Take the blocks in front of you and place them so that each of your forearms are resting comfortably on the blocks and you are gently lifting your shoulders and chest off the mat, your neck long and your gaze just past your fingertips.
3. Breathe gently here. You may notice your abdominals and back are engaged even though it is a supported posture.
4. If you would like to add something you can take your legs off the floor too, but that is totally optional.
5. Stay here as long as you are comfortable before moving the blocks to the side and bringing your arms in front of you, rest your head on your hands, totally relaxing your whole body.

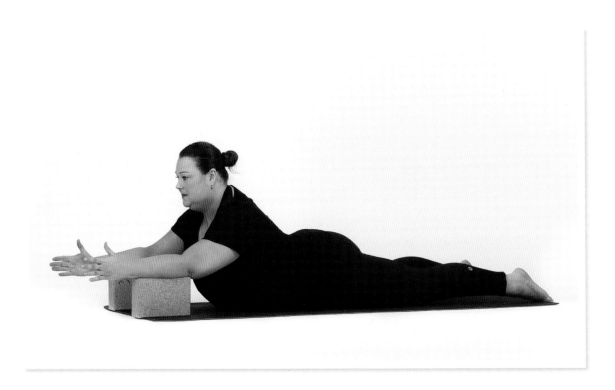

### Sphinx Posture – Salamba Bhujangasana

1. Lie on your front and come up onto your elbows so they are just under your shoulders or a little in front of your shoulders.
2. Your hands and fingers are pointing directly in front of you and lift your chest a little while relaxing your shoulders and face.
3. To stabilize your pelvis, tuck your right toes under and lift your right leg moving it backwards an inch or two before untucking the toes and repeating on the left side.
4. You may like to push back into Child's Posture (pages 84–85) as a lovely counterpose.

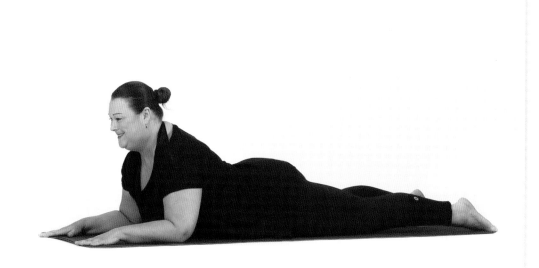

**Sphinx Posture version 2**

1. Lie on your front with your bolster across the mat in front of you, moving it so it sits mid-chest (or under your breasts, if you have them!).
2. Bring your elbows over the bolster so they are resting just in front of it with your forearms and hands pointing forwards.
3. To stabilize your pelvis, tuck your right toes under and lift your right leg moving it backwards an inch or two before untucking the toes and repeating on the left side.
4. Lift your chest and slightly tuck your chin in so your neck is in a lovely, long line.
5. Breathe here for 5–10 breaths, or this pose is suitable for a long hold.
6. You may like to push back into Child's Posture (pages 84–85) as a lovely counterpose, especially if you take a longer hold.

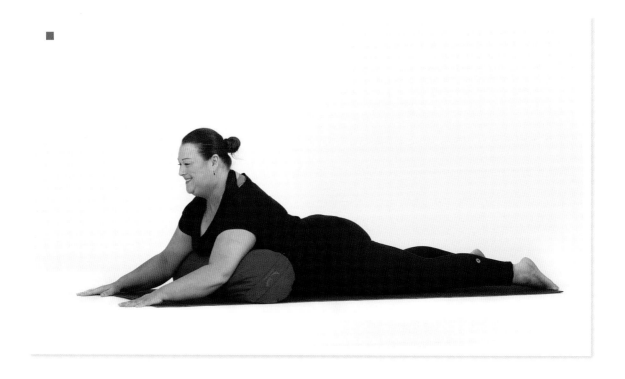

### Cobra – Bhujangasana

1. From the Sphinx or Crocodile Posture draw your hands, palms down, under your shoulders and take your feet to hip distance apart.
2. As you inhale raise your head, shoulders and chest up off the mat as you straighten your arms (do not lock your elbows).
3. Keep a bend in your elbows and gently draw them closer in towards your body. Tuck your chin slightly as you breathe here for 3–7 breaths.
4. Come back down to the floor and bring your arms in front of you, resting your head on your hands.
5. Bending your knees and lifting your heels towards the ceiling you can drop your feet to the left and right slowly (like a windshield wiper motion) to release your spine.
6. You may like to push back into Child's Posture (pages 84–85) as a lovely counterpose.

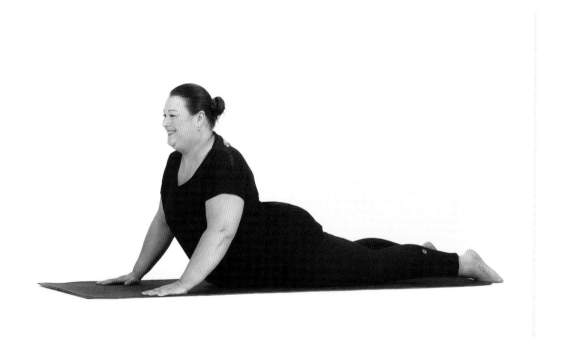

## INVERSIONS: WHERE YOUR HEAD IS LOWER THAN YOUR HEART!

### Downward Facing Dog – Adho Mukha Svanasana

1.  From Tabletop Position (page 72), move your hands a little further in front of your shoulders, if they are not already, and spread your fingers.
2.  Tuck your toes under and inhale and lift your hips up high and back slightly, firming your abdominal muscles.
3.  Keep a small bend in your elbows and knees to protect your joints (if it feels better, bend your knees to where your hamstrings feel more comfortable).
4.  Move your chest back towards your thighs so your ears are roughly in line with your inner arms (don't try this if it doesn't feel right for your body).
5.  Breathe here for 3–7 breaths then bring your knees back to the floor, sink your heels towards your buttocks, widen your knees and stretch your arms in front into Child's Posture (pages 84–85).
6.  If you like, come back to Tabletop and repeat.

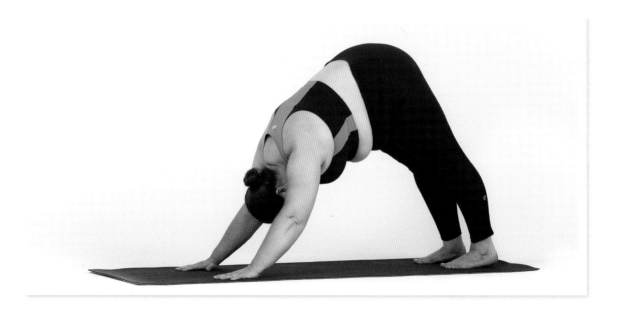

## Wall Dog

This posture can also be great using a chair instead of a wall, however I have included the wall version so that if you take a regular studio class without chairs you will know how to adapt Downward Facing Dog in any class!

1. Stand about a leg's length from the wall and, folding forward from your hips, bring your hands to the wall, about shoulder height (feel free to adjust for comfort).
2. Keep your knees soft and bend and sink your head and chest a little lower than your arms.
3. Breathe here for 5–10 breaths before bending your knees deeply, dropping your arms to your side and slowly coming up.

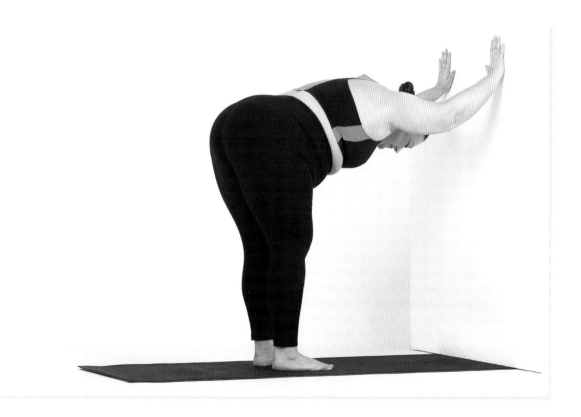

**Supported Shoulderstand – Salamba Sarvangasana**

When I say in class 'let's do a shoulderstand' there is sometimes a ripple of shock that runs through the class! The classic version can be quite tough, but this is lovely and restorative and suitable for most bodies.

1. Lie on your back with your bolster close by and bending your knees to hip distance apart, press into your feet and lift your hips into the air as you grab the bolster and place it under your hips (if this is tricky, asking the teacher or anyone at home to help shove the bolster under you is a good idea!).
2. Lift your feet off the floor and straighten your legs, feet pointing towards the ceiling.
3. You can flex your toes towards your face or leave them relaxed, and you can have a bend in your knees if you like, whatever is comfortable.
4. Keep your arms by your side with palms facing up or down and close your eyes.
5. Breathe here for 5–10 breaths and enjoy the benefits of going upside down in a safe way!

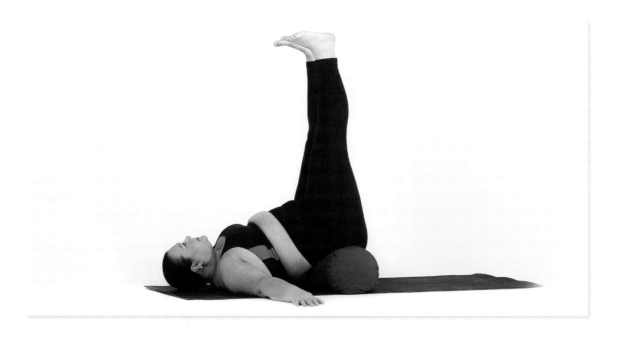

**Legs up the Wall – Viparita Karani**

1. Sit on the floor, scoot yourself as close as you can to a wall (facing sideways) with your knees bent up.
2. Gently lower yourself onto your elbows as you ease your torso to the floor and swing your legs onto the wall, legs at hip distance apart, with your heels on the wall.
3. Bring your arms out to the side and have your palms up or down, relax here and breathe for as long as you like!

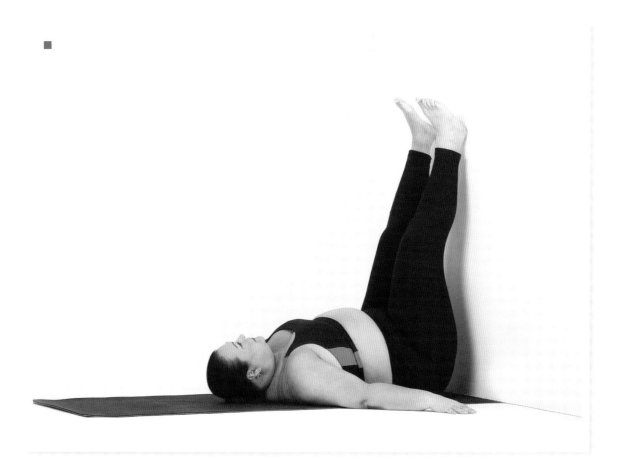

### Half Handstand – Adho Mukha Vrksasana

A stronger inversion, only suitable if you have no wrist or shoulder issues or injuries.

1.  Stand about a leg's length from the wall facing away from it.
2.  Fold forward and place both your hands on the floor, under your shoulders and take one leg up behind you to find the wall, pressing your foot firmly into the wall for support.
3.  Take the other foot to the wall and relax your head and neck. Make sure not to lock your elbows, keep them a little soft.
4.  Breathe here for 3–7 breaths and then gently step one foot to the floor followed by the other and return to standing.

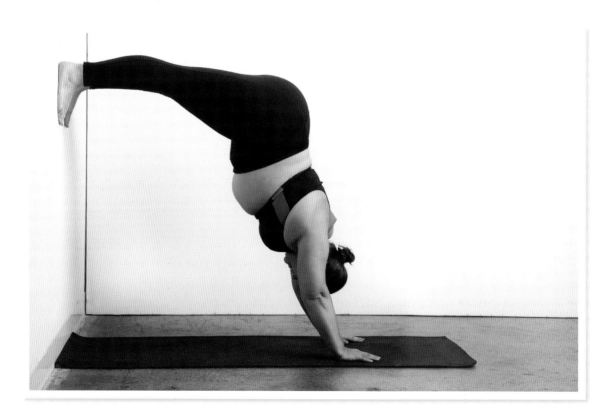

## RESTORATIVE POSTURES

This is the practice I go to when I am stressed, anxious or need to wind down for sleep. The best way I can describe it is delicious and nurturing. These postures can be practiced together or just one at a time (throw one into your regular practice to soothe your nervous system). Restorative Yoga is the antidote to our busy lives; the place to go when you are feeling overwhelmed and need a gentle and calming practice. I think it might just be my favorite!

Hold times: you can hold these postures for as long as you like! This practice is designed to be done in a sequence, if you like, and if you held each one for 7–10 minutes, it would be about an hour of restorative yoga. Go for it! You many never go back to any other kind of practice!

Props: Gather everything you have close by and make sure you are warm and comfortable. On hot days I sometimes use a sarong instead of a blanket as it gives the feeling of being wrapped up without being too stifling. I also really love an eye bag here (it puts a little pressure on the vagus nerve too, signaling the body to relax even further). Mine all have lavender and linseed…mmmm…delicious!

### My mind wanders, what do I do?
Minds are designed to think, worry, chat, comment and criticize! In the restorative postures sometimes that becomes more evident as we still our body and rest. Try to practice self-compassion; it can be a tricky to be still and come home to yourself and your body if it's an unfamiliar experience.

First, check in with yourself 'what do I need today?' and make sure you honor how you are (mentally and physically); perhaps you just need to let you mind wander today. Or maybe you need to bring your attention to the breath (sometimes I tell my students they can watch the rise and fall of the breath by noticing 'I am breathing in, I am breathing out').

### Restorative yoga and mental health
I am a trained and registered psychotherapist and I know yoga can be a key tool to support our mental health and also for healing. More and more research is emerging to support this, particularly with regard to restorative yoga (I suggest Bo Forbes's book *Yoga for Emotional Balance* for more information).

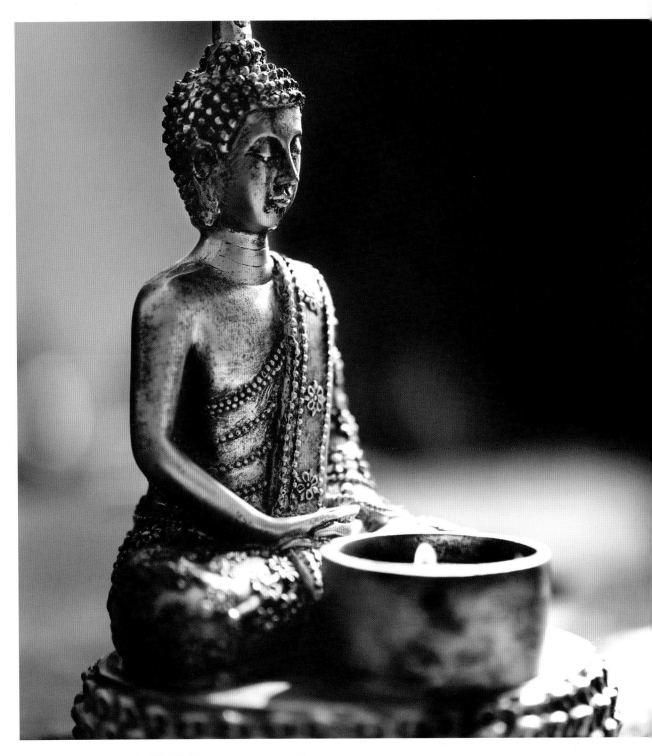

In the quiet stillness of this practice we come home to the body and become more aware of the landscape there. However, this can include low mood or anxiety or other body image worries, which can sometimes feel a bit overwhelming. In those cases, I suggest people seek help from practitioners who are both mental health clinicians and yoga teachers for support and bear in mind the idea of 'feeling' into the edges of the emotion so as to not become overwhelmed. Becoming more 'Interoceptive', or learning to sit with and recognize these strong emotions is a key part of healing and these practices are suitable for most, but if you find they aren't for you, that is fine!

Emotional awareness is a good thing! If you find you notice sensations, emotions or things come up for you that you weren't expecting, it can be a powerful and positive thing. In my yoga classes I often notice tears can come up in the still postures, and that is absolutely OK! (If I see I will sneak a tissue into your hand.)

Just allow yourself to notice the emotion and know that, like all thoughts and emotions, it will pass. Sometimes, although it seems unlikely, the yoga mat is a place of healing and processing. Sometimes it's the only time we slow down enough to reach inward and really connect with our experience of having a body, not just living from the shoulders up!

**Queen Posture**

1. From a seated position arrange your bolsters (or couch cushions!) with one across the top of your mat and the second on top of the first lengthways (making a sort of 'T' shape).

2. Bring yourself so the base of your spine is touching the end the bolster, legs out in front of you.

3. Ease yourself down onto the bolsters and grab a blanket or eye bag (or nothing!) and then decide on your leg position.

4. If your lower back isn't totally comfortable, keeping your knees bent and feet flat on the floor is advisable, but you can also choose to have the soles of the feet together (as pictured) or crossed legs (make sure to cross them the other way half way through).

5. Now you just relax! Palms up or down, breathing gently here for 3–10 minutes.

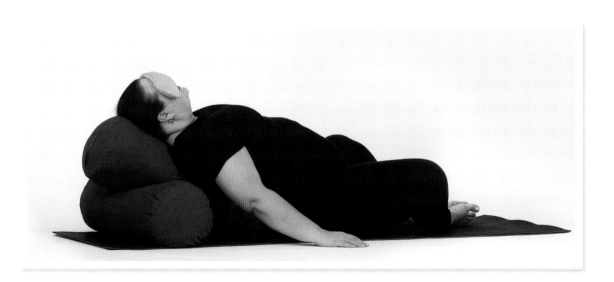

### Restorative Child's Posture

1. From a seated position arrange your bolsters in a similar way to the Queen Posture, however you are facing towards the bolsters here.
2. Bring the end of the long bolster under your pelvis (or if you prefer, onto your lower belly, this depends on the length of your torso).
3. Gently lower yourself onto the bolster and bring your arms around in front of the bolster, across the top of your mat, rest your head and torso on the bolster, totally supported.
4. Adjust your knees so they are about as wide as the mat (you can also pad them by placing a blanket under them).
5. I love placing a blanket over my shoulders (pictured) but you can wrap yourself up (or not) how you prefer.
6. And exhale! Stay here breathing gently for 3–10 minutes.

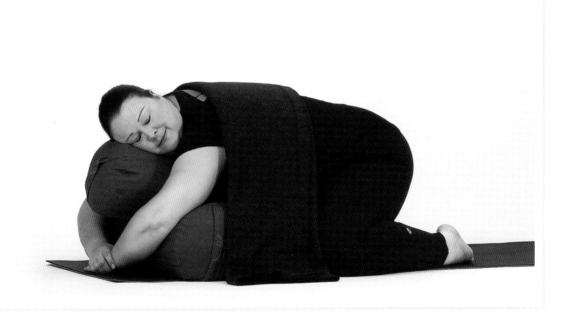

**Stonehenge**

1. From a seated position grab two blocks (or books of a similar size) and one bolster to build yourself a structure.
2. Place the blocks at about the width of your hips at the bottom of your mat (facing lengthways and whichever height you like) and then place the bolster over the top of the blocks, making what looks like a little Stonehenge structure!
3. From here bring your bottom towards the bolster with knees facing to the side of the mat and gently lower yourself to the floor as you swing your legs around to place them on your 'Stonehenge' at hip distance apart.
4. You can use your eye bag here or wrap a blanket over you, whatever feels good and you can have your palms up or down.
5. Enjoy and breathe for 3–10 minutes.

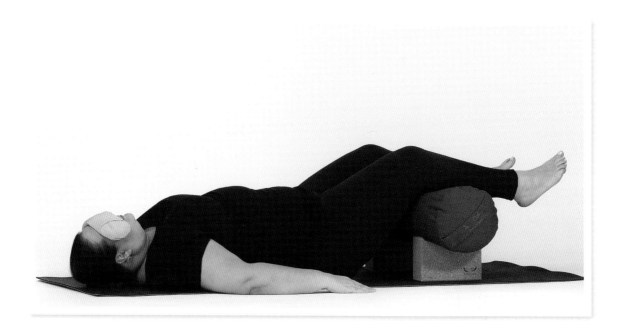

**Restorative Bridge Posture**

1. You only need one bolster for this delicious backbend; place it lengthways on the mat (in about the center) and sit on the edge of it with knees bent at hip distance apart.
2. Slowly lower yourself down onto the bolster so your head and shoulders rest on the mat (this depends on your range of movement, experiment with just having the head on floor if that seems more comfortable but be careful of your neck; you may even like another blanket under your neck).
3. Rest here with your palms up and breathe gently for 3–7 minutes.

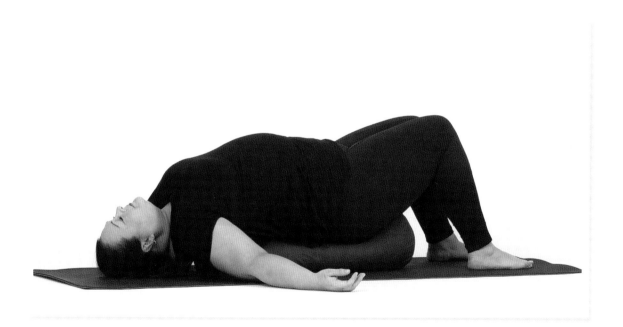

**Restorative Legs up the Wall**

1. From seated on the floor, scoot yourself as close as you can to a wall (facing sideways) with your knees bent up (have a bolster nearby).
2. Gently lower yourself onto your elbows as you ease your torso to the floor and swing your legs onto the wall, over your hips.
3. Bend your knees and if you would like a blanket to cover you, you may like to tuck it around your toes now.
4. Press your feet into the wall as you lift your hips as high as you can and bring the bolster under your hips (the bolster is flush to the wall or just an inch or two back).
5. Lower your hips on the bolster and then straighten your legs.
6. Your heels are on the wall, about hip distance apart and yours hands are on the floor, palms up or down.
7. I love an eye bag here. Breathe gently for 3–10 minutes.

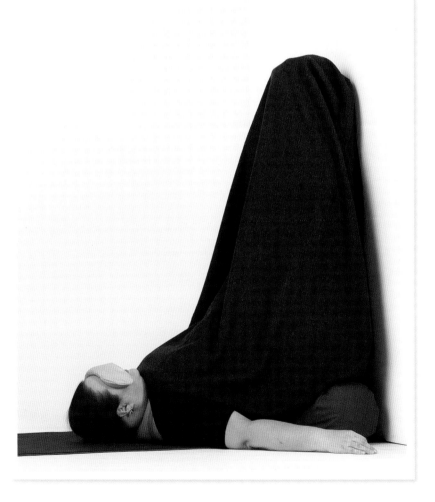

**Posture of Surrender – Savasana**

You can use this version of Savasana anytime!

1. First, make your neck roll (which can be used in any of the restorative poses) by folding the blanket so it's about as wide as your shoulders and then roll up about a quarter of the blanket, with the remainder facing away from you. Place it at the end of the mat.

2. Place the bolster under your knees and a blanket over your body and lower yourself onto your back with the neck roll supporting your neck.

3. Let your feet fall gently open and have your arms at a comfortable distance from your body, palms up or down.

4. Grab the eye bag last, if you like it, and begin the meditation on page 142 or lie in silence for 7–10 minutes as you enjoy the final posture, the posture of letting go.

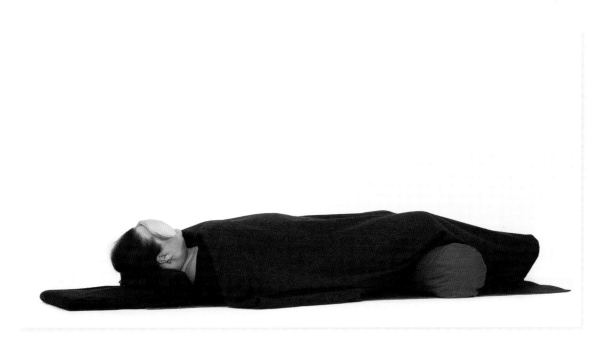

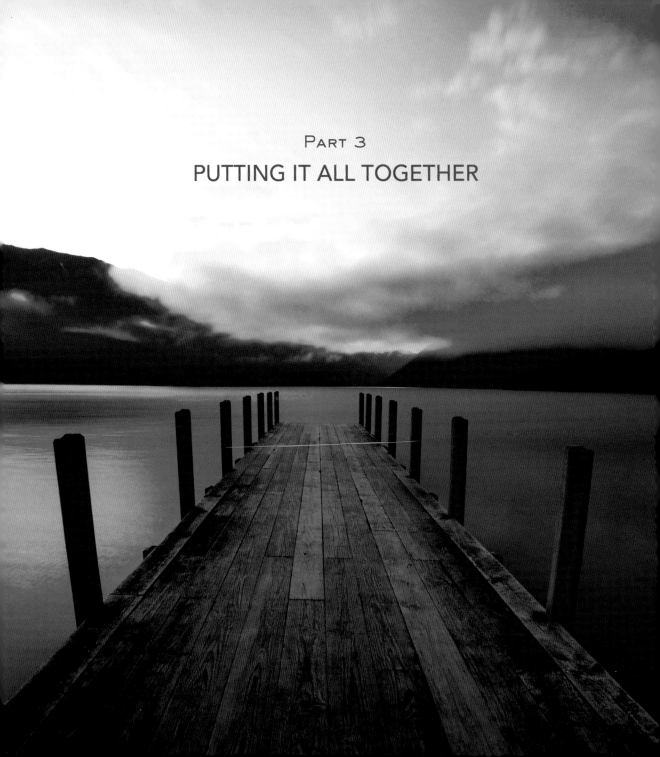

PART 3

PUTTING IT ALL TOGETHER

## CENTERING AND MEDITATIONS

I begin each class the same way, with some mindfulness, some self-compassion and a 'centering' practice to ready myself or my class to get the most out of the yoga practice.

Here is the script of what I usually say, which lasts about 5 minutes, usually before we start to warm up.

### CENTERING MEDITATION (you can record your own voice to listen to)

We will begin by lying down, so bring yourself into your most comfortable lying position (or if that is not available to you, remain seated) maybe with a bolster under your knees and something under your neck; you want to feel supported. You may close your eyes or leave them open.

Let's just take three 'sigh breaths' to release any tension by taking a deep breath in through the nose and 'sighing' it out through the lips. You might like to imagine you are breathing in a sense of calm and breathing out any worries or stress.

Now just give yourself a moment or two to notice you are here. You may like to reflect on your energy levels or any emotional tone you feel in your body, making sure that you adjust your practice to take into account those things.

Taking a short mindfulness pause to notice and observe how your body feels supported by the floor, observing the temperature of the air, any scents or sounds around you, the gentle rise and fall of the front of your body.

Taking a moment to acknowledge that you made space for yourself to show up on your mat today, which is an act of self-care and perhaps noting to yourself any intention you would like to make for this practice. If nothing comes to mind you can perhaps use this: 'I appreciate my body just as it is, even for a moment or breath or two.'

Feeling into the body and taking a moment or two to sense into the following five points; sensing into the left and right heel and the left and right palm and all the sensation there and then finally into the back of the head as it rests supported.

Remember, in this practice we honor the body. Taking care to be aware of our range of motion and respecting it. No forcing or straining and there should be no pain. Always look for a modification or move out of the pose slowly if it's not right for you.

Let's take a few yogic breaths before we move into the practice.

Begin by drawing your breath deep into the bottom of your lungs (your belly rises) then mid-lung (the side ribs expand outwards and upwards) and finally we bring it into the upper lung (the shoulders and collarbones moving up slightly).

A short pause before beginning to exhale; top lung, middle lung, lower lung.

Repeating a few rounds of this deep, slow, soothing breath before letting it go and letting the body's natural breathing take over.

## SAVASANA MEDITATION (you can record your own voice to listen to)

Savasana is the posture of surrender. Surrender of the body to the floor and perhaps surrender or slowing the thinking mind as we find this space of conscious relaxation and letting go.

Just noticing now too how your body is positioned and how you feel today. Your legs and feet can gently fall out to the side. Your arms are by your side, at a comfortable distance from your body, palms up. Make sure you are feeling no areas of tightness or discomfort and close your eyes when you are ready (if you feel happy with closed eyes).

Take a deep breath in and out through your nose and allow your attention to focus on the breath for a moment as you notice it settle, slow and fall into a natural rhythm. Feel how cool the air is as it moves through your nostrils and notice the temperature as it returns out of your nose. Then let the attention on the breath drop away as you let the body breathe naturally.

As you lie here you know there is nowhere else you need to be, that this is time you have to yourself to completely relax so begin to let yourself fold into your inner world and notice that your heart rate and your breath begin to drop down.

Remember that it's normal and natural for our minds to keep moving...and for thoughts to pop into our minds moving us away from this practice and somewhere into the future or the past. This is completely normal. It's how our mind works...just gently and without judgment thank your mind and allow it to return to the beautiful practice of Savasana or even just the breath or the feeling of your body supported by the floor.

Let's take a trip around the body...starting with your feet, bring your attention to your feet...let the floor support the feet...they are warm and heavy...relax your feet. Now, your ankles and calves...feel them relax and soften. Notice the small space under your knees...relax your knees and move your attention to the top of your thighs and then the bottom of your thighs...let the floor have the legs...soft and warm. Notice your pelvis relaxing and your buttocks sinking into the floor...no tension, soft and warm and supported. Your lower back eases and softens, melting into the floor. Bring your attention to your stomach and how it gently rises, softly, gently with the breath. Feel your upper back and shoulders...sinking...soft and warm, supported. Now your head, completely relaxed and your face and jaw eased and holding no tension with your teeth a little apart...Your whole body relaxed and calm, soft and melting...completely relaxed. Let the floor have the body...and your mind, let it become spacious too...allow any thoughts which bubble up to gently move along. It's totally normal for our mind to be busy...just allow this time as an opportunity for letting something else unfold inside us...let the business of your mind fall away and become more spacious and calm.

A few minutes of silence here...

It's lovely to have this time to ourselves, to be calm and turn inward, relax and consciously rest our nervous system.

Bringing your attention back to the sound of my voice...slowly moving our minds first and perhaps noting how this relaxation was for you today. All days are different, some easier to let everything fall away than others.

Gently...listen to the sounds we can hear just outside and how the blanket feels as it covers you, perhaps the temperature of the air around you.

When you feel ready you can activate more awareness, being kind and gentle in awakening yourself, you have been deep in relaxation.

Notice your breath, moving slowly in and out. Its own rhythm. You may like to deepen the breath slightly, moving more oxygen though your body. Slowly, gently, in your own time.

You may like to move your toes, your fingers, noticing how this feels.

At your own pace, you may like to gently stretch and point your legs, then do the same with your arms. If it feels comfortable, allow your body to stretch as if you were waking up...bringing your hands above your head and stretching your whole body.

Allow your eyes to open and adjust to the light in the room. We are going to very slowly and without words roll on our right side for a moment or two and then gently lift ourselves into a seated position. Take your time. There is no rush.

## BREATHING PRACTICES: PRANAYAMA

I encourage my students to find their own rate of breathing and I always incorporate some breath, or pranayama, practice into my class. It's also a fantastic skill to have in everyday life and while sometimes I don't get to my mat daily, I never go a day without some kind of pranayama practice, even a minute or two!

'Prana' means 'life force' or 'energy' in Sanskrit (very roughly translated, it is a complex idea in yogic philosophy) and the actual practices are called pranayama. Here are a couple of my favorites and there are many hundreds more if you would like to deepen your study of this 4000-year-old traditional practice.

### The Yogic Breath

Sit or lie comfortably and relax your whole body. It's often a great idea to start to learn this breath lying down so you can feel how the breath moves into each part of the body. We breathe in and out through the nose, if that is available to us, as it's another signal to the body that things are calm and relaxed.

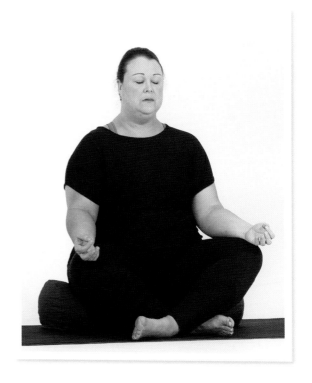

Begin by drawing your breath deep into the bottom of your lungs (your belly rises) then mid-lung (the side ribs expand outwards and upwards) and finally we bring it into the upper lung (the shoulders and collarbones moving up slightly).

A short pause before beginning to exhale; top lung, middle lung, lower lung.

Repeating a few rounds of this deep, slow, soothing breath before letting it go and letting the body's natural breathing take over.

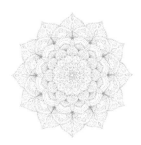

**'Sigh' breath**
Sit in your most comfortable position and take a long and deep inhale through the nose, then 'sigh' out the tension through the mouth (make as much noise as you like!).

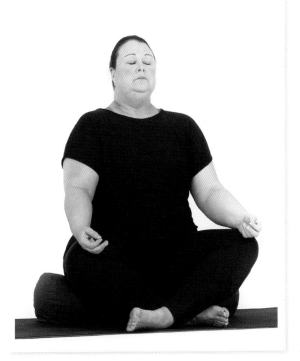
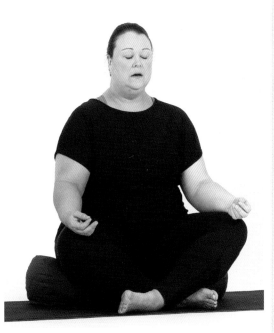

### 'Anxiety' Breath

Sit or lie and begin with your hands gently closed. As you inhale slowly and deeply, uncurl your fingers at the rate of your breath, stretching your fingers and hands away from you (strong stretch through the fingers). As you exhale long and slowly, you bring your fingers back to fists, tightly squeezing them.

This breath helps both through the deep and even breathing, but also by the stretch and clench of the hands, releasing anxiety and giving the mind something to focus on. If you want to use this breath in a public place you can always practice it with your toes! That way no-one can see!

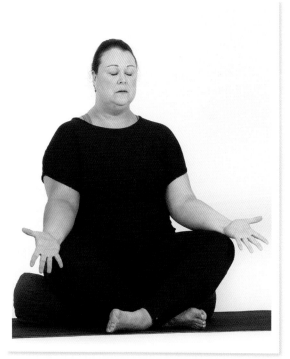 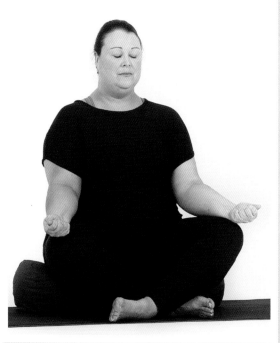

### 'Joyous' Breath

I am a bit of a nerd and I love neuroscience! One of the fun facts about the brain is that it can't tell the difference between a real smile and a fake one and the brain will still release some great hormones and endorphins with a fake smile.

This breath is adapted from the work of Amy Weintraub. It can be used anytime, but I like to use it to shift my mood or if I am feeling in a bit of a funk or anxious.

Sit in your most comfortable position and, with open or closed eyes, take a long, slow inhale through the nose and as you exhale, smile and drop your chin to your chest. Inhale, lift your chin and repeat!

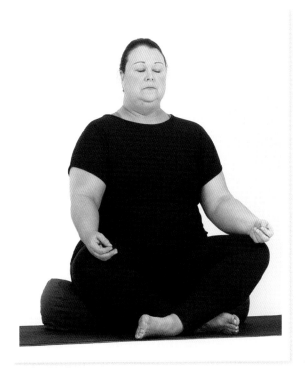
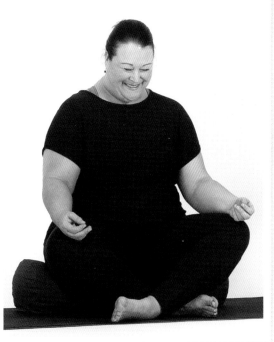

**'Heart Opening' Breath**

I often use this breath as part of my warm-up (after the Seated Salute page 44) and it's a great morning breath. Bring your forearms together in front of you with your hands together in Anjali Mudra (just pressing lightly together). As you inhale, slowly take your arms back as far as they can comfortably go behind you, keeping them at shoulder height and lifting the chest and drawing the shoulder blades together with palms facing out to the sides. As you exhale, bring your forearms back together. Repeat as many times as you like.

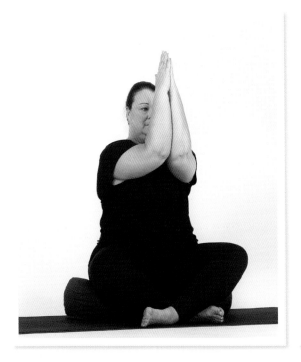 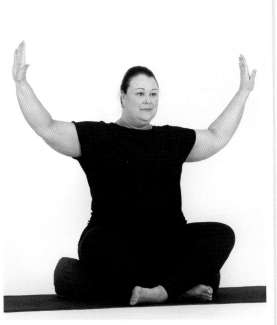

## MUDRAS

Mudras are symbolic hand positions or 'seals' used in yoga (and also in many Eastern wisdom traditions). In yoga we use these hand gestures, often while seated, to seal the 'prana' or life-force in, often in conjunction with pranayama.

There are many mudras but I have chosen my favorites and the ones I teach and practice the most often. I find them calming, almost like a signal to myself that I am now sitting to practice my meditation or yoga, not just sitting playing on the floor with the dog!

### Gyan Mudra – The Mudra of Knowledge
Sitting comfortably, bring your hands to your knees with palms up and your thumb lightly touching your index finger. This is one I use for sitting and meditating or just gentle pranayama.

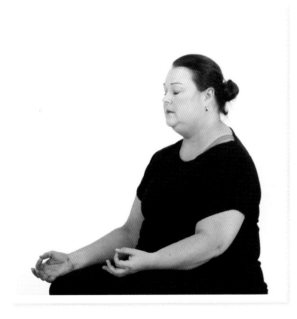
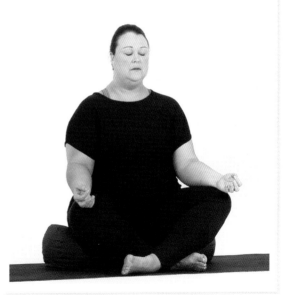

**Anjali Mudra – Prayer Position**

Bring your hands together at your heart, lightly pressing together with your thumbs resting on the middle of your chest. This is the mudra I use to begin or close a class. I was taught it as a reminder that your practice is a form of prayer or offering to yourself. I find it peaceful and grounding and it is a good mudra to use when you would like to set an intention for your practice.

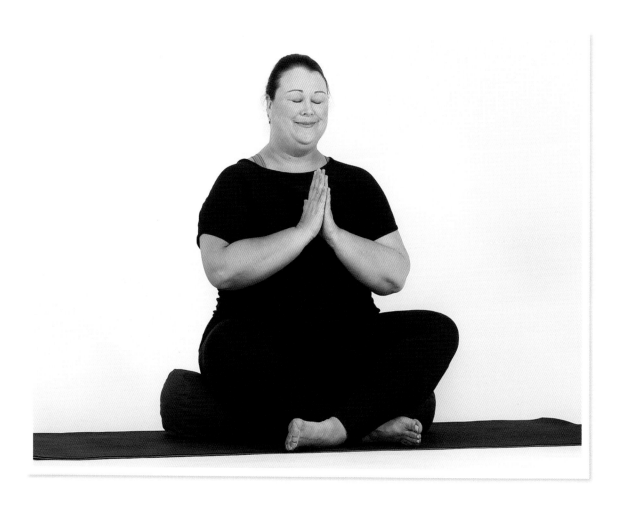

## Lotus Mudra

Bring your hand together at chest height, just in front of your body. Connect the heels of the hands and gently touch the fingers, a little space between them. As you inhale, open your fingertips out (thumb and little finger stay connected) and as you exhale come back to the first position.

In Buddhism the lotus blossom represents a heart opening. The lotus flower blooms on the surface of water, with its roots deep below in mud and the lotus is a symbol that even in mud, beauty can flourish. I have always been very attracted to this mudra and I often wear jewelry with the lotus flower on it.

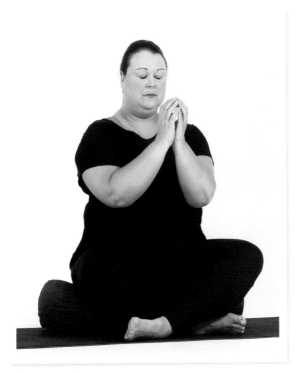 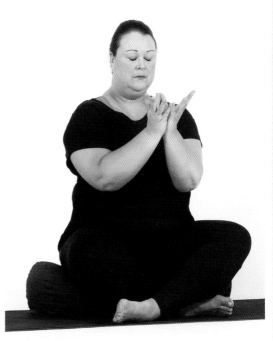

### Garuda Mudra – Eagle Mudra

Linking your thumbs with one hand on top of the other, stretch out your fingers like wings and place your hands on your heart. For me this is the mudra of self-compassion. Every time I practice it I send myself love and gratitude. Or if that feels too hard some days, I just repeat to myself 'may I be safe, may I be loved, may I be happy' (a Metta, or loving kindness, meditation).

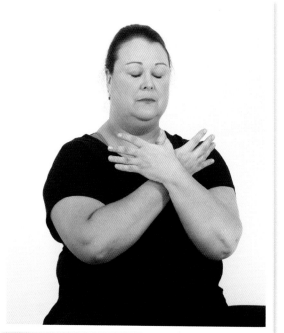
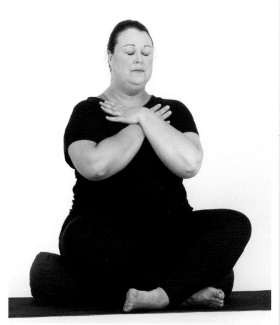

## CREATING A HOME PRACTICE

You are ultimately the person who will decide which postures you do and how long you practice for! Here are some ideas for how to structure your practice and I would advise doing some warming of the body every time you practice.

To put together your own practice, use the 'arc' outlined on page 32 and pick some postures from each group after you have warmed up. I suggest the following go later in your practice for safety:

» Head to Knee posture (page 70)
» Wide Leg Forward Bend (pages 95–96)
» Pigeon (pages 81–83)
» Sphinx (pages 123–124)
» Camel (page 78)
» Locust (pages121–122)
» Triangle (page 87)
» Half Handstand (page 130)

### Warm-up
Begin with Centering (page 141)
Then use the seated Salute to the Sun x 2–3 (page 44)
Cat/Cow x 5 (pages 73–74)

### 10–15 minutes to practice
Savasana for a couple of minutes to center your mind (pages 118–119 )
Seated Salute to the Sun x 2 (page 44)
Cat/Cow (pages 73–74) x 5
Tiger x 2 (page 75)
Downward Facing Dog x 3 (page 126)
Mountain Posture (page 86)
Tree Posture (page 103)
Swan Dive (page 99)
Sphinx (pages 123–124)
Extended Child's Posture (pages 84–85)

Lying Twist (pages 111–114)
Savasana, for as long as you have! (pages 118–119)

**60-minute practice: classic self-compassion class**
Centering, 5–7 minutes (page 141)
Knees to Chest (pages 115–117)
Seated Salute to the Sun x 3 (page 44)
Cat/Cow x 5 (pages 73–74)
Tiger x 3 (page 75)
Modified Wild Thing x 2 (page 76)
Child's Posture 5–10 breaths (pages 84–85)
Tabletop (page 72)
Downward Facing Dog x 3 (page 126)
Eagle Posture (pages 104–105)
Warriors 1 and 2 (pages 91–92)
Swan Dive x 5 and hold the last one as long as you like with head down (page 99)
Half Moon Posture (page 106)
Sphinx (pages 123–124)
Child's Posture (as a counterpose to the backbend) (pages 84–85)
Seated Twist (page 69)
Eagle Mudra with yogic breath
Wide Leg Forward Bend (pages 95–96)
Knees to Chest (pages 115–117)
Lying Twist (pages 111–114)
Any version of Bridge Posture you fancy (pages 108–110)
Legs up the Wall/Supported Shoulderstand or Half Handstand (pages 129, 128 and 130)
Savasana (10 mins) (pages 118–119)

**60–75 minutes: restorative yoga to soothe and calm (pages 131–139)**
Centering, 10 minutes (optional)
Restorative Queen Posture, 10 mins
Restorative Child's Posture, 10 mins
Restorative Stonehenge, 10 mins

Restorative Bridge, 6–8 mins
Restorative Legs up the Wall, 10 mins
Restorative Savasana, 10 mins

**Finishing your practice**
I usually bring everyone to their most comfortable sitting position with their hands in Gyan Mudra. Close your eyes if you like and take three 'sigh' breaths. Then take your hands to Anjali Mudra and take a couple of breaths, letting a word rise up inside you to describe how you feel right now and just tuck that away. You may also like to take a moment to be with yourself in gratitude. You made the time to show up for yourself in self-care, which is sometimes not easy to do.

*May I be safe (thumbs between your eyebrows, palms together)*
*May I be loving (thumbs on your lips, palms together)*
*May I live with ease (hands at your heart in Anjali Mudra)*
*May I accept myself as I am (Anjali Mudra)*

(Buddhist Metta Meditation)

Namaste.
I hope you enjoyed your practice.

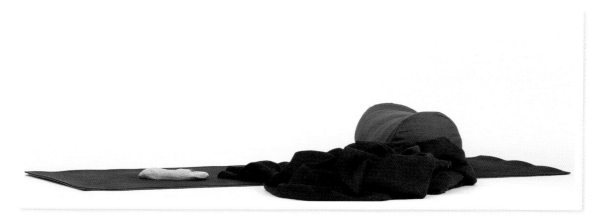

## MEDICAL DISCLAIMER

The information provided in this book is for educational purposes only. All exercise involves a risk of personal injury, and you should consult a medical practitioner before commencing any new exercise program, including yoga, to ensure that you do not injure yourself.

Practicing under the direct supervision and guidance of a qualified yoga instructor may reduce the risk of injuries. Not all yoga poses are suitable for all people. Please seek the advice of a qualified yoga instructor or your medical practitioner to help determine which poses are suitable for you.

If you feel dizzy, light headed, faint or if you experience any other discomfort, stop exercising immediately and consult a medical practitioner. Exercise within your limits. Never force or strain. Seek attention and advice as appropriate.

## ABOUT THE AUTHOR

Sarah Harry is a leading body image and eating disorders specialist and offers a unique perspective as an experienced clinician, lecturer, researcher, yoga teacher and writer. Sarah has practiced yoga for more than 20 years, is the owner and founder of Fat Yoga and runs specialist classes and retreats. She is also co-director of Body Positive Australia alongside Fiona Sutherland.

Sarah is a member of the Yoga and Body Image Coalition (USA), sits on the National Advisory Board of HAES Australia and is a member of the National Eating Disorders Coalition.

## ACKNOWLEDGMENTS

**Photoshoot credits**
Lucia Ondrusova you are the best, you went above and beyond and it was a pleasure to work with you to create such amazing pictures! The activewear is by Sonsee Woman, it was a dream to wear! Thanks Vanessa (and Janine for the hand delivery). The clothes in the lifestyle shots and cover were generously provided by 17 Sundays and Alison Dominy Designs. Thank you Ashleigh Carpenter for the hair and make-up and Malabella for the special mala. A special thank you to Stretch Now who provided all the props and then donated them to my yoga hospital program, you are so kind. Finally, a huge thanks to Anahata Giri at One Heart Yoga and Meditation Studio for letting us use your studio for the photoshoot.

**I offer my gratitude to all these wonderful professionals, family, friends and students:**
To all my students, present and past, you inspired me and taught me more than I can ever express, your support of Fat Yoga humbles me. The people who keep showing up to class are the heart of this movement. To my kids, Max and Charlie, I love you more than you could know. Thank you to my parents Mary and John, there are no words to express all you have done for me. All my incredible family and friends, you are there for me in so many ways I am grateful for and I love you so dearly. Much love to the 'Moist Women' and my 'Magic Tribe', you know who you are. To Emily D for the push to start doing it differently.  To Janet, Nadine, and Karen for answering my yoga questions with grace and Emma, Pip and Fiona for their reading and feedback. Thank you to the studios who rent me space, without you we wouldn't be able to do this.

A massive thank you to everyone at New Holland who helped bring this book to life: Fiona Schultz, Lorena Susak, James Mills-Hicks, Liz Hardy and Jessica Nelson, you have all been incredibly patient and supportive. To Monique Butterworth, thank you for seeing a book in my pitch and for saying 'yes'!

To the following clinicians, yogis and activists who I have never met, but who have inspired and taught me so much: Brené Brown, Kristen Neff, Linda Bacon, Anna Guest Jelly, Dianne Bondy, Connie Sobczak, Judith Hanson Lasater, Virgie Tovar, Cyndi Lee, Bo Forbes, Melanie Klein, Melody Moore, Suzie Orbach, Amy Weintraub, Donna Farhi and BKS Iyengar. Masters all.

First published in 2017 by New Holland Publishers Pty Ltd
London • Sydney • Auckland

The Chandlery 50 Westminster Bridge Road London SE1 7QY United Kingdom
1/66 Gibbes Street Chatswood NSW 2067 Australia
5/39 Woodside Ave Northcote, Auckland 0627 New Zealand

www.newhollandpublishers.com

ISBN: 9781742579313

Group Managing Director: Fiona Schultz
Publisher: Monique Butterworth
Project Editor: Liz Hardy
Designer: Lorena Susak
Production Director: James Mills-Hicks
Printer: Hang Tai Printing

10 9 8 7 6 5 4 3 2 1

Keep up with New Holland Publishers on Facebook
www.facebook.com/NewHollandPublishers

US $25.00
UK £16.99